The Natural Healing

·ANNUAL·

1987

The
Natural Healing
·ANNUAL·

1987

Edited by
Mark Bricklin
Executive Editor, PREVENTION® Magazine

Written by the Staff of Rodale Press

 Rodale Press, Emmaus, Pennsylvania

ISBN 0-87857-680-0   hardcover

2 4 6 8 10 9 7 5 3 1   hardcover

Contents

Nutritional Healing Newsfront

New Frontiers in Vitamin and Mineral Research: 1987 Update

Friendly Fats

Cosmic Nutrition for the Inner You

"Feel-Better" Foods

It's an "off day" for your health and your appetite but you need to keep nutritional strength on "high." Do you force yourself to eat? No! say our experts, and give better recommendations. 60

Nutritional "Boosters" for Your Middle Years

Top researchers are saying a lot of what we accept as normal "aging" problems are really nutrition problems. (Learn why one major health center is looking to see if extra vitamin E can "energize" the immune system.) 65

The Vegetarian Edge

Something about the vegetarian lifestyle seems to promote health and keep away problems like diabetes, gallstones and even more serious conditions. 70

The Super Health Power of Omega-3

It reduces cholesterol and triglycerides and makes dangerous blood clots less likely. It can relieve arthritis pain and headaches. In lab animals, it helps block tumors. For you and me, it can also make a great gourmet dinner! 75

Is Your Body Too Dry?

Dehydration doesn't only come from sweating buckets. Common medications, for instance, can dry you out—especially dangerous for older folks! Among the early symptoms are weariness, impatience and dizziness. 82

Bioelectrical Healing Report

Sometimes the body needs to be "jolted" into healing an old injury. Scientists can now do the job painlessly, and say this new approach may "revolutionize the practice of medicine" in coming years.............. 196

Stress Control Reports

Stress Patrol: How to Spot a Sneak Attack

Poor concentration, too many colds, digestive upsets, insomnia, backaches, a long list of common complaints may be secret signals that your circuits are carrying too much "high-tension" current................. 203

First Aid for Your Feelings

Feeling burned out? Left out? Nervous? Disappointed? Use these quick-learn tips to smooth your feathers and start flying high again. 211

Busy Person, Calm Mind

Just because you're a high achiever doesn't mean your wages must include worry, tension and turmoil. Here's the latest approach used to help restore tranquillity to the frazzled. 218

A Gun Called Stress

It can get you right through the heart. To keep heart attack at bay, consider two things: what's been going on in your mind; what's been going into your mouth. 225

A Good Talk Is Good Medicine

When medical treatment doesn't clear up a youngster's chronic condition, suspect stress. Often, a good confidential talk can uncover the cause and lead to rapid relief.. 231

Weight-Reduction Bulletins

Health on the Home Front

How to Arrive Alive

SUPPLEMENTS AND COMMON SENSE

Some of the reports in this book give accounts of the professional use of nutritional supplements. While food supplements are in general quite safe, some can be harmful if taken in very large amounts. Be especially careful not to take more than these commonsense limits:

Vitamin A	20,000 I.U.
Vitamin B_6	50 mg.
Vitamin D	400 I.U.
Selenium	100 mcg.

NOTICE

The information and ideas in this book are meant to supplement the care and guidance of your physician, not to replace it. The editor cautions you not to attempt diagnosis or embark upon self-treatment of serious illness without competent professional assistance. An increasing number of physicians are ready to cooperate with clients who want to improve their diet and lifestyle; if you are under professional care or taking medication, we suggest discussing this possibility with your doctor.

Introduction
1987: A Year for
Regeneration

A friend of mine in California went to his doctor and was told that his blood pressure was creeping up. Usually around 130 over 90, it had, in the space of a year, bubbled up to 144 over 94.

"Lose some weight," the doctor said. "You're about 25 pounds over what you should be, and that could be the problem right there."

But my friend had always been 25 pounds overweight, and his paunch had never been blamed for anything other than spoiling his profile.

"Is this old age?" he asked me. "Does old age start at 42?"

That's a good question. I was thinking about it just last night when I saw Paul McCartney in a video and noticed that his hair was turning gray.

Three days ago I spoke to my friend Dick again. It had been just about 10 months since he told me about his blood pressure.

"So how's it doing?" I asked.

"How's what doing?"

"The blood pressure."

"Oh, that. No problem. Down to about 124 over 84. In the morning, it's about 118 over 80, then goes higher. Peaks when I get home after driving on the freeway and then starts going down again."

"How do you know all that?"

"Oh, I bought one of those home pressure units. The digital kind. It's fun."

"Well, how did you get your pressure down?"

"Honestly, I'm not sure. I did just about everything. Lost weight, for one thing. Dropped from 190 to 169. No desserts, only two drinks a day, no pizza for late-night snacks. And exercise, too."

"Like what?"

"Started with jogging. Killed myself on these hills out here. So I tried swimming but I got tired of it and started walking the hills instead. Two-and-a-half miles a day, in 40 minutes."

Dick went on and on, about his exercise, the calcium pills he was taking, the fruit he ate and the meditation tapes he listened to for 15 minutes before walking each day. That's why he said he really didn't know *what* had lowered his pressure. All he knew was that it was lower than it had been for ten years, and that he felt "fantastic."

His mother, he added, had said to him "and think of all the money for drugs you saved!" To which he'd answered, "Mom, if you knew how much I just paid for a new wardrobe, you'd get sick!"

Although Dick didn't have a specific name for what he'd done to chisel down his body and blood pressure, here at *Prevention*, we do. We call it Regeneration.

At 42, Dick was in no way wallowing in old age. Rather, he'd forgotten to keep in touch with his youth. Eventually, it began to sort of . . . wander off, and the first sign of "old age" came to fill the vacancy. Dick's all-around program of good habits literally regenerated his youth and his health.

Regeneration. The simplest way to think of it is as self-improvement. Improvement *of* the self, *by* the self. Calling on your own resources, biological, psychological and spiritual, to restore vigor and purpose that seem to be flagging. And sometimes, you come up with rewards that seem to be brand-new territory. A feeling of zest for life, for instance, that you haven't enjoyed since you-can't-remember-when.

Besides all those new health habits, Dick did something else that can be called regenerative: He went to his doctor regularly for checkups. Now, not all medical care can be called regenerative in a meaningful way. Taking pills to calm your nerves may be necessary, but it doesn't *restore* anything. It merely mollifies and masks. Kind of like putting a bucket under the leak in the roof. Disaster is prevented but the problem remains. It may even get worse if you're content to put out more and more buckets—or take more and more tranquilizers.

Medical care that gives you an early warning of trouble can be regenerative, though, if you and your doctor use that information to begin rebuilding health.

I'd even call certain kinds of surgery regenerative. Implanting an artificial hip, for instance, can open the door to a whole world of healthful activity that would otherwise be impossible to the victim of an accident or severe arthritis. Surgery that restores vision is another good example. A not-so-good example? Coronary bypass might qualify, because it doesn't halt the progress of arterial disease, and its effects don't last very long. It can reduce angina pain, certainly, and so may be necessary— even wise. But it can't be the whole answer, only part of an answer that includes major lifestyle improvement—regeneration, in other words.

Your 1987 *Natural Healing Annual* is packed with information you can use to help move your own regeneration program ahead. The emphasis is on what you can do for yourself, now. But the medical aspect is here, too. No longer is there a big, dark canyon between prevention and natural healing on one side, and medical services on the other. Regeneration has bridged that gap. An important part of prevention is proper medical checkups, while progressive doctors are more and more prescribing natural healing techniques for body and mind.

Still, regeneration remains something you must ultimately do for yourself. No one can eat for you, not even the world's greatest nutritionist. No one can exercise for you, not even the greatest coach. No one can sleep for you, or smile for you. Nor can anyone go to the doctor for you, ask questions for you, take medication for you . . . or be optimistic for you. Or, for that matter, read this book for you.

That's why all health care is ultimately self-care.

Mark Bricklin
Executive Editor
PREVENTION® Magazine

Nutritional Healing Newsfront

New Frontiers in Vitamin and Mineral Research: 1987 Update

Scientists continue to probe vitamins and minerals trying to learn more about the nutritional supplements and looking to add to the list of already known benefits. Within the past year or so, vitamin and mineral intake or therapy has been studied in relation to hearing loss, infertility, premenstrual stress syndrome, depression, diabetes and cancer, among other maladies. What follows are some of the more noteworthy developments of late.

Vitamin A

The ancient Greeks deduced that eating certain foods would cure night blindness, although it wasn't until 1913 that vitamin A was identified as the reason. The professor who unraveled its chemical structure won a Nobel Prize almost 20 years later, and scientists have been hot on the case of vitamin A ever since.

Most recent interest has focused on beta-carotene, which is found in many green and yellow fruits and vegetables. Beta-carotene turns to vitamin A in the body and scientists have been toying with the theory that the compound may inhibit cancer. That premise gained credibility when a five-year study of dietary habits among the elderly revealed that those with diets high in green and yellow vegetables were less likely to get cancer.

A team that included scientists from Harvard Medical School and Boston University followed the eating patterns of more than 1,200 people over the age of 66. They came away unable to state with certainty that the vitamin A component was the protective agent, which wasn't necessarily a defeat, since they did suggest that "some factor" may be providing the effect. Their conclusion: "Even in old age, higher intakes of green and yellow vegetables are still associated with lower risks of cancer death" (*American Journal of Clinical Nutrition,* January, 1985).

Meanwhile, investigators in Italy formed a similar conclusion. They reported in the *International Journal of Cancer* that women whose diets were high in carrots and green vegetables were less likely to get cervical cancer.

It's probably safe to assume that the potential of vitamins will continue to pique the curiosity of the scientific community. For instance, there's a hint of a chance that folic acid may help with behavior problems that come with some forms of mental retardation; vitamin E might alleviate the noncancerous lumpy breast tissue that plagues up to 20 percent of the women in the United States; vitamins A and C may help modify the risk of smoking and alcohol consumption in the development of mouth and throat cancer, and initial evidence suggests children who get enough vitamin A might avoid some types of lung or digestive problems.

In the meantime, most scientists would probably agree that the words "cautiously optimistic" could best describe the attitude as they continue their efforts. And those M.D.'s and Ph.D.'s who are fond of clichés could employ a well-worn one in this case: nothing to lose and everything to gain.

Stay tuned.

Vitamin B₆

Clinically, the condition is referred to as carpal tunnel syndrome, but to those who suffer with the swollen fingers, the stiffness, numbness and tingling in their hands, relief is more important than labels. The usual treatment is anti-inflammatory medication or cortisone injections to reduce swelling. If the drugs fail, surgery is recommended, which sometimes doesn't relieve the pressure on the median nerve that's causing the problem. Vitamin B_6, a member of the B complex family, may offer some hope.

The connection between B_6 and carpal tunnel syndrome has been a topic of heated debate within the research community for years. Recently, Britain's medical journal *Lancet* fanned the embers by reporting the successful use of B_6 to treat carpal tunnel syndrome.

A West Coast neurologist has thrown even more tinder to the B_6 fire. Allan L. Bernstein, M.D., chief of neurology at Kaiser Hospital, Hayward, California, has found that 150 milligrams a day brings improvement in three to four months, with the daily dosage dropping to about 25 milligrams after six to twelve months. "It took longer for the older patients to respond because their systems had to be resaturated with B_6 and their degree of compression was greater, whereas the younger ones had a less severe injury and responded in a shorter amount of time," he says.

While there have been no side effects from the dosages, Dr. Bernstein cautions that excessive B_6 can be toxic and cause neurological problems. (Don't take more than 50 milligrams a day without medical guidance.) He advises that people who suspect they are suffering from the syndrome discuss B_6 therapy with their physician, especially if more drastic measures— particularly surgery—are suggested.

Besides the physiological stiffness, B_6 may also help emotionally, a conclusion that emerged during carpal-tunnel research, says Herman Baker, Ph.D., a professor of preventive medicine, community health and medicine at the New Jersey Medical School, Newark.

"We know that a lack of B_6 is linked to depression, although we still don't understand how it all works," Dr. Baker says. Doses of 100 to 200 milligrams have proved successful so far. "The important thing for a person suffering from chronic depression to realize is that taking supplemental B_6 will not alone correct the problem. B_6 must be part of a total program that includes other factors, like changes in lifestyle." Medical guidance is needed for the large doses of B$_6$ used by Dr. Baker.

A New Role for Biotin

The vitamin biotin plays a major role in the synthesis of fatty acids and the metabolism of glucose—often called blood sugar. These processes are faulty in people with diabetes. Those two facts led several researchers across the country to investigate a connection between biotin and diabetes.

Studying tissue and blood samples of a group of insulin-dependent diabetics, the scientists found the diabetics had far higher tissue levels of biotin than normal subjects, although their blood levels of that nutrient were about the same.

The significance? High levels of biotin in tissue are related to increased levels of blood sugars, or glucose, a serious factor in diabetes.

On the other hand, increased blood biotin levels caused blood sugars to drop—and that is exactly what happened when these diabetics took biotin daily for a week.

Therapeutic doses resulted in a hundredfold increase in the biotin levels of their blood, and glucose levels fell off significantly as well.

The researchers aren't precisely sure why this happened, but they speculate that in diabetics, biotin may be abnormally bound and thus unavailable for use in the body (*Annals of the New York Academy of Science*, June 24, 1985).

Folic Acid

Around 70 million adults, or 40 percent of the total adult population, take vitamins each day, and most probably aren't aware of the folic-acid content in the tablets they swallow. What sounds like something that would eat through your clothes is actually a B-complex vitamin that helps the body manufacture red blood cells and is essential for converting food to energy.

It's long been known that a deficiency causes a type of anemia, but now it appears that low levels of folic acid may be linked to lung cancer caused by cigarette smoking.

Scientists at the University of Alabama, Birmingham,

have found low levels of folacin in the blood of cigarette smokers who developed abnormal cells in the bronchial lining.

The researchers are attempting to pinpoint whether smoking affects folic-acid levels in the bronchial lining itself, making conditions favorable for the onset of precancerous conditions (*American Journal of Clinical Nutrition,* April, 1985).

Vitamin C

Multiple vitamins aside, the most popular single vitamin is still C, or ascorbic acid. Of the almost $2 billion in total over-the-counter vitamin sales in 1984, almost 20 percent was for vitamin C. Part of the reason is that man, like guinea pigs and like other primates, can't synthesize vitamin C within the body and must depend on external sources.

Scientists previously have shown that ascorbic acid may increase resistance to infection and protect against some environmental pollutants. Smokers and women taking birth-control pills are believed to be at risk of vitamin C deficiencies.

There have also been suggestions that C helps ward off cancer. That claim has been reinforced by Australian scientists who found that high intakes of vitamin C reduce the risk of rectal cancer, according to preliminary information from the Australian Society of Epidemiology.

Several thousand miles away, a report in the *Scottish Medical Journal* indicates vitamin C helps lower levels of hazardous LDL cholesterol in elderly men. The research was promoted by the theory that the low levels of vitamin C often found in the elderly might in some way be tied to increases in LDL cholesterol that also occur in the later years. They found that one gram of C daily reduces LDL cholesterol levels by as much as 15 percent (*Lancet,* October 20, 1984).

Back in the United States scientists at the University of Texas, Galveston, have increased male fertility with vitamin C. Men with infertility problems caused by sperm clumping together and not moving freely were given one gram of vitamin C daily for a month. After three weeks the clumping decreased dramatically, and total sperm count more than doubled.

"All of the subjects were deficient in vitamin C when they came in," says E. B. Dawson, Ph.D., of the school's obstetrics and gynecology department. "But before anyone goes popping vitamin C in hopes of improving their fertility, he should first find out what's causing his problem. There are a variety of reasons for a man to be infertile and they all can't be corrected with vitamin C."

Vitamin D

Everyone needs vitamin D for strong bones and teeth, and women who are postmenopausal and susceptible to osteoporosis need it more than others. But vitamin D may also have implications for cancer, diabetes and hearing loss.

Vitamin D comes from sunshine and some foods, and is converted by the liver and kidneys into its active form, a hormone called calcitriol that regulates the calcium balance in the body. Research in Japan has found that the hormone suppresses leukemia cells by causing them to be turned into noncancerous cells.

"Where this will go therapeutically isn't clear at this stage," says Hector DeLuca, Ph.D., director of biochemistry at the University of Wisconsin, Madison. "In the long run, someday we may be able to control some types of leukemia. This may also have applications for controlling other types of malignancies."

Dr. DeLuca's own research also suggests that a vitamin D deficiency may lead to problems with glucose metabolism and, ultimately, insulin secretion. "Part of the falloff in glucose tolerance that occurs in many older people could be due to a lack of vitamin D, so if we can prevent the deficiency of calcitriol, perhaps we can control some cases of diabetes."

There's also a chance that a form of hearing loss associated with the cochlea, a tube shaped like a snail shell that forms a crucial part of the inner ear, can be prevented. Apparently the cochlea needs vitamin D and calcium just as much as the skeleton and teeth. When a deficiency occurs, minerals and hearing slowly fade. So far, hearing has been restored in some cases with daily supplements of calcium and 500 to 1,000 international units (I.U.) of vitamin D. Refer your physician to the *Journal of Laryngology and Otology,* pp. 405-420, May, 1983.

Preventing the hearing condition or catching it in the

early phase is essential, since the deafness may be reversible. Just as important is that early detection could point to the onset of osteomalacia, a bone-degenerating condition, before more serious skeletal problems occur.

As if the case for getting out in the sunshine wasn't strong enough, a study spanning almost two decades found that men who developed colorectal cancer had lower intakes of vitamin D and calcium. A research team of scientists from across the country discovered that those men who developed cancer also weighed more and got less exercise than those who remained free of the disease, which "supports the suggestion that physical activity is inversely associated with the risk of colon cancer" (*Lancet,* February 9, 1985).

Older Skin Needs Its Day in the Sun

As your skin ages, vitamin D plays hard to get. And a vitamin D deficiency can lead to dangerously soft or brittle bones.

Researchers aren't sure why, but the skin of young people appears to be a more efficient vitamin D factory than the skin of older adults. As skin ages and becomes thinner, it becomes less productive at turning out vitamin D from sunlight, according to a recent study.

To prove the point, scientists took skin samples from a number of surgical patients. The patients ranged in age from 8 to 92. Each sample was bathed in ultraviolet light—similar to the UV in sunlight. When they checked the samples, they found that young skin produced the most vitamin D. In the older, thinner skin samples, vitamin D production decreased in proportion to the age of the individual. The skin of one 82-year-old produced less than half the amount of vitamin D churned out by the 8-year-old skin (*Journal of Clinical Investigation,* October, 1985).

How much sunlight does older skin need to make enough vitamin D? "That's almost impossible to say precisely," says Michael F. Holick, Ph.D., M.D., director of the Vitamin D and Bone Metabolism Laboratory at Tufts University. Dr. Holick was one of the researchers in this study. "It depends on so many things—skin pigmentation, time of year, location and so on. But we can say this: If, say, you're in Boston in June at noontime, you should expose your hands, face and arms, 15 minutes at a time, two to three times a week. In the winter, you'd probably have to expose a much larger area of the skin for a much longer period of time because the sun's rays are much weaker. In this case, vitamin D supplements are a desirable alternative," he says.

Dr. Holick suggests taking 400 I.U. of vitamin D daily. That's the Recommended Dietary Allowance for vitamin D, he says, and that should be all otherwise-healthy older adults need to take to supplement their diet.

Vegetarians and Rickets

The elderly aren't the only people who need vitamin D. Everyone needs vitamin D for strong bones, but not everyone gets enough. Among the most vulnerable are vegetarians, whose diets don't always provide sufficient vitamin D. Additionally, the high percentage of roughage in a vegetarian's diet may interfere with the absorption of this important vitamin.

Consider, for example, the severe deficiencies reported by researchers in Norway among vegetarian children. Several children in that country were hospitalized for rickets, or osteomalacia, a disease characterized by progressive bone softening.

These children also may have been predisposed to rickets because of the vitamin D-deficient diets of their vegetarian mothers, according to researchers.

After they were diagnosed, the children were given vitamin D supplements, and the painful symptoms of rickets disappeared altogether (*Acta Paediatrica Scandinavica,* volume 74, 1985).

Vitamin E

There's now evidence that E helps reduce premenstrual stress symptoms that make the time of month unbearable for some women. Scientists in Baltimore at Sinai Hospital and Johns Hopkins University School of Medicine found that 150 to 600 I.U. of vitamin E reduces a number of PMS symptoms, including nervous tension, mood swings, irritability, anxiety, headaches, craving sweets, fatigue, dizziness, fainting, depression, forgetfulness, crying, confusion and insomnia (*Journal of the American College of Nutrition,* volume 3, 1984).

How the vitamin relieves PMS troubles is uncertain, but one theory holds that E may affect levels of androgen, a hormone that's been linked to moodiness and depression.

Finnish researchers have noted an improved sense of well-being in elderly people who took vitamin E and selenium, which they speculate may protect cells from oxygen damage and slow the aging process. Although they used mammoth doses of both, they report no side effects. They did note improvements in anxiety, depression, fatigue, hostility, anorexia, mental alertness, self-care, motivation and initiative (*Biological Trace Element Research,* May, 1985). Further research needs to be done in this area before anyone can self-administer the large doses used here.

A Side of Bacon with Vitamin E

The federal government has approved a product that could make bringing home the bacon a little healthier.

Both the U.S. Department of Agriculture and the Food and Drug Administration have approved the use of alphatocopherol, a form of vitamin E, as an optional ingredient in bacon to inhibit the formation of cancer-causing chemicals in the cured meat. Called nitrosamines, these chemicals are formed when sodium nitrite, added to bacon to prevent botulism, combines with amine compounds in the meat during cooking. Vitamin E helps prevent this reaction.

The Agriculture Department has ordered manufacturers to limit the levels of nitrites in bacon, and routinely tests the fried product for the formation of nitrosamines, known to cause cancer in animals. Though there are more nitrosamines in secondary cigarette smoke and smokeless tobacco—one researcher calls it the "ubiquitous carcinogen"—bacon has the highest level among cured meats.

The first vitamin E-enhanced bacon is expected to appear on grocers' shelves soon. Alphatocopherol is to be listed as an ingredient. This product will have been either injected with or dipped in a salt brine containing alphatocopherol. In addition, the FDA has approved the use of a spray product developed by Hoffmann-LaRoche, a vitamin manufacturer.

The vitamin E-treated bacon won't taste any different nor is it expected to cost much more, about a penny per pound.

But the process should reduce nitrosamine content in the fatty part of the meat by 70 to 80 percent, according to some estimates. Manufacturers already add ascorbic acid, or vitamin C, to bacon to inhibit nitrosamines in the lean portion of the meat.

Calcium Lowers Blood Pressure—The Evidence Mounts

A new study from doctors at the Oregon Health Sciences University, in Portland, reinforces previous findings that high intakes of calcium lower blood pressure. David A. McCarron, M.D., and Cynthia D. Morris, Ph.D., gave 1,000 milligrams of calcium a day for eight weeks to people with high blood pressure and people with normal blood pressure. For the sake of comparison, they also gave them a placebo for another eight weeks.

They found that calcium significantly lowered blood pressure in the patients with hypertension. Forty-four percent of them achieved a reduction in systolic pressure (the higher number) of ten points or greater. The people with normal blood pressure remained essentially unaffected by taking additional calcium. The placebo had no significant effect on either group.

"Treatment with 1,000 milligrams per day of oral calcium for eight weeks represents a safe, well-tolerated, [nondrug] intervention that lowers blood pressure in selected patients with mild to moderate hypertension," they conclude (*Annals of Internal Medicine,* December, 1985).

Of particular interest is the doctors' observation that calcium's blood-pressure-lowering effect seems to be time-dependent—the pressures really began to drop only after six weeks. "A trial shorter than eight weeks might have failed to show an effect, whereas an even greater response might have occurred if calcium was extended beyond eight continuous weeks," they say.

Latest Theory: Salt Fights Calcium

As if there weren't already enough reasons to take the saltshaker off the table, there's new evidence that sodium may play a role in calcium loss.

Ailsa Goulding, Ph.D., senior research officer, department of medicine at the University of Otago, in New Zealand, believes that consumption of common table salt increases the amount of calcium lost through the kidneys. In one study, animals given salt supplements lost more calcium and phosphate—another element in bone—in their urine and had less of the minerals in their skeletons than those animals not receiving salt. Another study found that adding a teaspoon of salt to the daily diet of young women increased the amount of calcium lost. Dr. Goulding also found that a single teaspoon a day can cause enough of a calcium loss to decrease bone mass 1.5 percent a year.

The relationship between salt and calcium excretion may be one reason why women in primitive societies that add no sodium to food suffer less bone loss than U.S. women, even though their calcium intakes are low by our standards. It may also help explain the relationship between low calcium intake and high blood pressure in countries with high salt consumption, such as the United States.

Early Milk Drinking: Will It Prevent Bone Loss?

Here's another argument to try on your kids when they won't drink their milk.

Scientists at the University of Pittsburgh have found that drinking milk during childhood and adolescence may reduce the risk of postmenopausal osteoporosis, a bone disease that causes over 148,000 hip fractures a year and has a mortality rate of 12 to 20 percent.

The researchers came to this conclusion after examining the lifetime milk-drinking habits of 255 white, upper- to upper-middle-class women, ages 49 to 66, who were in menopause for at least a year.

The women who recalled drinking milk with every meal as children and teenagers had higher bone densities than those who drank it less frequently. They also tended to have a higher calcium intake at their current age than women who had drunk less milk, though the study also indicated mean calcium intake of the participants was, in general, low.

The researchers suggest that such early intervention—

that is, more milk drinking in childhood—may impart some protection against the ravages of later bone loss (*American Journal of Clinical Nutrition,* August, 1985).

Aluminum Pots? Stop Worrying

Dietary aluminum has been a topic of debate in research circles for years. Some scientists claim the metal can lead to a variety of problems, including Alzheimer's disease. But curb your anxieties if you fear that dangerous levels of aluminum from the pot are getting into the roast.

Researchers at the University of Wisconsin, in Madison, report that you probably get far more aluminum in your system from other sources than you do from food prepared in pots made of the metal.

During the Wisconsin project, the scientists cooked 26 different foods in aluminum and stainless-steel pans, disposable aluminum trays and aluminum foil. Some foods did indeed accumulate aluminum during cooking. Acidic foods, such as tomatoes and applesauce, showed a slight increase.

The key word here is "slight." A 100-gram portion (about half a cup) of tomato sauce, which is about one average serving, contained 5.7 milligrams more aluminum after cooking—the largest increase among the foods tested. Most adults probably consume 20 to 40 milligrams of aluminum daily through their normal, everyday diet (*Journal of Food Protection,* September, 1985).

Magnesium

● Much of the Western world doesn't get enough magnesium, and the result could be a higher incidence of heart disease and hypertension. That's because many areas are served by a soft-water drinking supply, which lacks the magnesium content of hard water. Magnesium plays a part in keeping your heart muscle beating rhythmically.

People living in hard-water areas may bemoan the fact that their soap won't lather as readily. On the other hand, the incidence of heart-disease-related death is 10.1 percent lower there than in soft-water regions, according to the journal *Magnesium* (vol. 4, no. 1).

Additionally, studies show a relationship between low magnesium levels and high blood pressure and stroke. Your muscles, bones, nerves and teeth also need this multipurpose mineral.

● Magnesium deficiency may adversely affect your ability to stand up to long periods of vigorous exercise.

At the University of California, at Davis, rats fed a magnesium-deficient diet ran out of gas faster than their brother rats, who consumed a normal diet—normal for rodents, that is. This research suggests that the rats' exercise capacity declined along with the magnesium in their diet.

It is far too soon to tell what impact this new research will have on humans. But studies are under way at Davis to explore the effects of magnesium deficiency on people. This continuing research could provide some insight into the impact of magnesium deficiency on the human immune system as well.

● People who attempt suicide may have low levels of magnesium in cerebrospinal fluid, according to research from the Regional Neuropsychiatric Institute in Hungary. Magnesium is thought to be necessary for the release of serotonin, a neurotransmitter that strikes a balance between manic and depressed behavior.

● In several studies, magnesium has been reported useful in controlling premature labor and fetal growth retardation. This doesn't apply to all expectant mothers, but to those at particular risk for premature delivery. It has been theorized that magnesium deficiency disturbs the delicate metabolism of the placenta (*Magnesium,* vol. 4, no. 1).

● Patients who receive radiation therapy for cervical cancer sometimes find that the treatment involves damage to the colon, leading to chronic diarrhea. Israeli researchers found that intravenous magnesium, along with antidiarrhea drugs, alleviated the diarrhea. They theorize that radiation decreases serum magnesium levels. In turn, diarrhea may be a result of magnesium deficiency.

Previous research has laid the groundwork for these provocative new theories.

"There's a lot more to this than just subjective ideas,"

according to Burton M. Altura, Ph.D., professor of physiology at Downstate Medical Center, in Brooklyn, New York, and founder of the American Society for Magnesium Research. "Now we have a lot of objectivity, a lot of good scientific work being done. This isn't to say that all these things will pass the test of time. But certainly, the cardiovascular aspects that have come to the forefront over the last five to seven years are valid and are going to be extremely useful in the diagnosis and treatment of patients with various types of cardiovascular ailments." Full-blown magnesium deficiency is not common in the West, says Dr. Altura. The problem, he says, is border-line deficiency.

"It's a serious problem," he adds. "The public must become aware of this and must attempt to have a balanced diet."

The Recommended Dietary Allowance for magnesium ranges from 300 milligrams for women to 350 milligrams for men. Nuts and whole grain cereals are good food sources of magnesium.

Copper

Some women who suffer frequent miscarriages early in pregnancy are low in copper. Recent research suggests a strong connection.

"This was a very serendipitous observation," says Maryann Breskin, a research associate in the department of nutrition at the University of Washington. "We were looking at something else—zinc and copper levels throughout pregnancy. We real-ized that some of these girls who were losing their babies sometimes had low copper levels."

Previous animal studies have established the relation-ship between zinc and copper and fetal malformation, Ms. Breskin says.

Copper helps your body absorb iron. Copper deficiency can lead to skeletal malformation and albinism. Also, the rare genetic Menke's disease, known as "kinky hair syndrome," results from a genetic inability to absorb copper. The mineral plays a part in fertility and in the formation of hemoglobin. Copper deficiency also has been linked to high serum choles-terol levels.

The National Academy of Sciences recommends from 2 to 3 milligrams of copper daily for adults, roughly half that amount for children. Nuts, seeds, red meats, liver and organ meats are good sources of this mineral.

Potassium

Researchers at the University of Minnesota Hospital and Medical School recently found that lab rats with high blood pressure had fewer fatal strokes when potassium was added to their diet. This, even though blood pressure remained about the same (*Hypertension,* vol. 7, no. 3).

That's fine for hypertensive rats, but what about people? This study suggests that increased potassium in the human diet could reduce the occurrence of potentially fatal brain hemorrhages.

Potassium also keeps your ticker in sync. Your pancreas needs potassium, too, in order to secrete insulin.

Fresh fruits and vegetables—bananas, tomatoes, celery, cabbage and grapefruit, to name a few—are excellent sources of potassium.

Zinc

High levels of stress may lead to temporary zinc deficiency. In one study, hospital patients awaiting surgery showed clinical signs of deficiency in the form of dermatitis. The rashes, scaly skin and ulcers responded well to oral zinc supplement and zinc oxide ointment (*Journal of Parenteral and Enteral Nutrition,* vol. 9, no. 3).

Zinc sulfate solutions may prevent oral and genital herpes. William W. Halcomb, D.O., of Austin, Texas, has reviewed recent research on zinc and herpes. He says the antiherpes claims appear to be accurate, although there still is no definitive cure. "Zinc either prevents or slows down multiplication of the herpes virus, for reasons not clearly understood," says Dr. Halcomb. "The lesions heal in a shorter time."

Zinc, it seems, truly is the nutrient of many faces, playing a role in the maintenance of male fertility, disease resistance, brain development and cell growth. It helps your gums resist the harmful effects of dental plaque. Without zinc in your diet, even your taste buds take a snooze. Food doesn't taste as good.

If you have a wound or burn, zinc helps it heal. Your skin needs zinc, too. If you see white spots on your fingernails, it could be a sign you aren't getting enough zinc. The RDA for zinc is 15 milligrams daily. Food sources include liver and beef. Popcorn, Cheddar cheese and peanuts are good sources, too.

Friendly Fats

Not all fats wear black hats. But we're not talking blubber here. We're referring to a variety of fats known in clinical circles as polyunsaturates, and they do indeed wear the white hats. Polyunsaturates may help prevent heart attacks by decreasing dangerous cholesterol and preventing clotting, which leads to heart attack and stroke. There's also evidence that polyunsaturates may play a part in lowering blood pressure. Scientists are just beginning to scratch the surface of their worth, with implications for arthritis, allergies, menstrual problems and possibly multiple sclerosis.

Invisible Fat

If anything, fat is familiar. It hides belts, it sits on the plate after being trimmed off the pot roast and it rests on kitchen shelves in the guise of lard and shortening. These are the visible fats. Yet, the majority of the fats we ingest are invisible and lurk in unsuspected places—Cheddar cheese and frankfurters, for example. Many of these are saturated fats, the nutritional villains that do so much damage.

For years various health organizations have warned of the dangers of too much fat in the diet, and advised lower levels. According to the American Heart Association, heart disease, stroke and related disorders kill almost as many people as all other causes of death combined.

The major underlying cause of these diseases is atherosclerosis, a buildup of fatty deposits within artery walls, which restricts and sometimes blocks blood to the vital organs. Studies implicate high cholesterol levels in the blood and high blood pressure as major contributors to atherosclerosis.

One of the easiest ways to clog arteries and raise blood pressure is to eat saturated fats, which usually originate in land animals—meat and full-fat dairy products, for instance. While the body needs some saturated fat to function properly, it can manufacture almost all it needs. The surplus we ingest just causes trouble.

Fat versus Fat

On the other hand, polyunsaturated fats, which usually come from vegetables, seeds, nuts and aquatic creatures, can displace the saturated fats and, in a sense, neutralize their negative effects. But this healthy blocking can only occur if the polyunsaturates outnumber the saturates, which, for most red-blooded Americans, is usually not the case.

Unfortunately, Americans are eating far more of the bad than the good. "In general, we're consuming 2½ times more saturated fat than polyunsaturated fat," says Jon Lewis, Ph.D., a pathologist at the Bowman Gray School of Medicine, Wake Forest University, Winston-Salem, North Carolina, who has conducted long-term studies on fats and human nutrition. "We know without a doubt that saturated fats do unhealthy things, such as drive up cholesterol levels, but people are still eating too much."

Ideally, roughly equal amounts of the two fats, along with another type called monounsaturated that has many of the same characteristics as polyunsaturates, should be the rule of thumb, a recommendation that resulted from the 1977 Senate Select Committee on Nutrition and Human Needs. That group also concluded that no more than 30 percent of a day's calories should come from fat; currently, we get about 40 percent.

When the Senate committee convened almost a decade ago, cholesterol was undoubtedly in the back of the members' minds. Today, it's in the public forefront, mainly because almost one million people annually die from diseases of the heart and blood vessels that are often the result of excess cholesterol.

The sad fact is that many of the deaths might have been prevented. As early as 1950 evidence surfaced that vegetable fats lowered cholesterol levels while animal fats caused an increase. In the ensuing years, more studies emerged reinforcing the theory. Yet, as with almost any facet of medicine, there are two sides to every story.

Two Sides to Cholesterol

"The important thing to remember is that we're talking about two kinds of cholesterol," says Richard L. Jackson, Ph.D., of the department of pharmacology and cell biophysics at the University of Cincinnati College of Medicine. "We're looking for a ratio of polyunsaturates to saturates that will lower levels of LDL cholesterol, which is the unwanted type, and maintain high levels of the beneficial HDL cholesterol. It's been shown that an extremely high polyunsaturate/saturate ratio will lower HDL levels."

Dr. Jackson and several colleagues found that it doesn't take radical shifts in the polyunsaturate/saturate balance to achieve some healthful effects. They concluded that a polyunsaturate/saturate ratio of one-to-one, rather than the harder-to-consume ratio of four-to-one used in previous studies, lowered LDL levels better while maintaining HDL.

Plugging the Pipes

While they still aren't sure how it works, researchers believe that polyunsaturates also decrease the risk of clotting in the bloodstream, which means less of a chance of a heart attack or stroke. One of the more popular theories is that the polys block the release of an acid in the cells that encourages clotting. Research so far has shown that diets high in saturated fats fill blood cells with this acid, priming the person for a potential clotting problem.

One source of polyunsaturates that's suspected of blocking this clotting acid is fish oil, which is gathering attention in scientific circles. West German researchers found that daily doses of cod-liver oil help prevent clumping of platelets, the chief characters in the clotting process. The supplemental fish oil also lowers thromboxane (a substance that causes clotting and vessel constriction, and increases bleeding times), another indication that clotting risk is eased (*Circulation,* March, 1983).

According to Leo Galland, M.D., and a growing number

of other experts, more fish should be in everyone's diet because they are high in a type of polyunsaturated fatty acid called omega-3, which keeps the harmful clotting factors from getting together. "Nationwide there's a deficiency in omega-3," says Dr. Galland, who has conducted research on the role of fatty acids on health and currently codirects a New York clinic specializing in nutritional medicine. "A majority of the population should increase their intake of omega-3. The best source is fish that live in cold climates, such as salmon, tuna, herring, sardines, even lobster and oysters. It's also in green, leafy vegetables and linseed oil, but not as concentrated as in fish."

Thar She Blows

Fish oil is also being touted as a way to lower blood pressure, a claim reinforced by that same West German study. The researchers found that the cod-liver oil lowered systolic blood pressure an average of almost ten points.

The strongest evidence that polyunsaturates lower blood pressure comes from a military base near San Francisco that houses the U.S. Department of Agriculture's Western Human Nutrition Research Center. There, research has shown that by increasing the polyunsaturated-fat intake from the current norm of 3 to 4 percent up to 6 to 7 percent of total calories, blood pressure may drop 10 to 15 percent.

Exactly how this happens is unclear, according to center director James Iacono, Ph.D., but the most plausible theory is that the good fats improve kidney function and cause more sodium and potassium, known contributors to high blood pressure, to be excreted in urine.

The most appetizing aspect of Dr. Iacono's research is that an easy-to-follow menu produces the desired results. "In the past two studies, we lowered blood pressure in 40- to 60-year-old men and women without reducing their intake of meat, dairy products or salt," he says. "You just have to use lean meats, low-fat dairy products and keep salt intake to the usual 8 to 12 grams a day."

One phase of the research was conducted in Finland, land of the highest death rate related to cardiovascular disease and the home of people who consume massive amounts of saturated fat. People on a low-fat diet emphasizing polyunsaturates showed dramatic blood-pressure reductions, whereas those on a low-sodium diet had only slight reductions, says Dr. Iacono.

Coexisting with Fat

Other scientists around the globe are just beginning to dabble with polyunsaturates, with some encouraging initial findings. Doctors in England report using a diet high in essential fatty acids to calm hyperactive children, and there are documented cases of polyunsaturates helping people who suffer from arthritis, allergies and multiple sclerosis.

While the research continues, the best approach is one of moderation. Says Dr. Lewis, "The biggest mistake people could make is to assume that radically increasing their intake of polyunsaturates will help even more. Fats are fats, regardless of the type, and you should cut back wherever possible. If you have to use a fat, make sure it's a polyunsaturate."

In general, only about 30 percent of daily calories should come from fat; of that 30 percent, at least 10 percent should be polyunsaturates to counteract the 10 percent saturated fats that you're bound to ingest.

The remaining 10 percent should be monounsaturates, the beneficial fats that were previously thought to be neutral. "Our initial research shows that monounsaturates may be just as effective at lowering blood cholesterol," says Fred Mattson, Ph.D., professor of medicine and former head of the lipid research clinic at the University of California at San Diego. "Monounsaturates may even be more beneficial because they don't lower HDL cholesterol levels like excessive polyunsaturates do. But people shouldn't worry about getting enough because a normal diet usually supplies all that are needed."

The best thing about all of the good fats is that they can be had without having to stare at a bland, lifeless dinner plate. Substitution is the word for the day.

"You can easily make subtle, what I call passive, changes in the way you prepare foods that may make a difference in long-range health," says R. Curtis Ellison, M.D., professor of medicine and pediatrics at the University of Massachusetts Medical Center, in Worcester.

The Ultimate Test

Dr. Ellison braved life and limb by trying his substitution theory on high-school students, and found that despite a few exceptions, the foods prepared with polyunsaturates passed the test.

"Many of the oils used in schools and for commercial food preparation are high in saturated fats. We wanted to see if using polyunsaturated products would be acceptable because if so, then it could make a big difference in the health of a lot of people who eat out in restaurants and in cafeterias at school or work," says Dr. Ellison.

The list of ingredients included safflower, sunflower and corn oils; margarine, cheese and salad dressings high in poly-unsaturates; potato chips fried in poly oil; even ice cream with a fat content that was 80 percent polyunsaturate. "With the exception of some commercially prepared meats, all of the products we used can be found on market shelves," he says. (The foods used in the USDA blood-pressure research were also grocery-store variety.)

Substituting skim for whole milk also helps, as does eating lean meat with all visible fat trimmed off, including removing chicken skin. When buying processed foods, label reading is advised, since some products—crackers and cookies, for instance—contain saturated fat to increase shelf life. Be particularly wary of items containing coconut or palm oils, two widely used and highly saturated fats.

Weight-loss programs should also be given a careful eye, since a diet may be devoid of the essential fatty acids that the body needs, Dr. Galland advises.

Cosmic Nutrition
for the Inner You

One of the best friends your bones ever had just traveled 93 million miles to get here. It's sunlight, and if you aren't outside welcoming it, well, maybe you don't know what you're missing. But your bones do.

The sun, that untiring nuclear furnace, brightens our days, warms our cold bodies and melts the snow. But the sun is more than just a pretty face. The sun's rays also trigger an ingenious biochemical process in our skin that stimulates the production of vitamin D, and that's good for our bones, too.

Get enough sunlight—just 10 to 20 minutes a day, experts say—and your skin will manufacture all the vitamin D your body needs.

Fortunately, most Americans get plenty of vitamin D. But a number of the nation's elderly—though no one knows exactly how many—live in the shadows, locked away from the light of Earth's shining star. As a result, their bodies don't make enough vitamin D. Neither do they get enough vitamin D in their diet, a secondary but important source of the vital nutrient.

Why is vitamin D so important? Think of vitamin D as a bus. Every day, calcium—an essential mineral—takes a ride on that bus. Its destination: your bones.

Calcium makes your bones strong and hard. Without calcium, your bones can become dangerously soft or brittle. But calcium has to have a way of getting from your gastrointestinal tract to your bones. That's where vitamin D comes in.

Vitamin D formed in the skin is converted in the liver to a prohormone, 25-hydroxyvitamin D. It's then converted once again in the kidney to an active hormone, 1,25 vitamin D, or calciferol. This hormone is what moves calcium along on its way to your waiting skeleton.

"The main thing vitamin D does is help the GI tract absorb calcium," says Patrick Ober, M.D., of the Bowman Gray School of Medicine, in Winston-Salem, North Carolina. "Calcium won't be absorbed and it won't ever be utilized unless it can be transported into the bloodstream, and that's the function of vitamin D."

Deficiency Can Be Crippling

Exactly how much vitamin D does the average person need? The Recommended Dietary Allowance of vitamin D is 400 international units (I.U.) daily.

Thanks to the sun, most of us get enough vitamin D without even trying. But for those who spend little time outdoors or cover up every available patch of sun-receptive skin, vitamin D deficiency can be both painful and potentially crippling.

In adults, prolonged vitamin D deficiency may lead to osteomalacia (soft bones) or osteoporosis (brittle bones). There's more to osteomalacia and osteoporosis than just a reduction in the amount of calcium going to your bones. Your body needs calcium for other purposes—to keep your heart beating rhythmically, to regulate muscle contractions, to promote blood coagulation and, in general, to keep your body's cells glued together. When your body doesn't get enough vitamin D, the bones don't get calcium, but neither does the rest of your body. So it responds to immediate calcium needs by siphoning calcium from the bones.

The early warning signs of osteomalacia are bone tenderness or pain, back pain, irritability and weakness. These symptoms often are dismissed as the inevitable consequences of old age. But it's not necessarily so. Left undiagnosed, osteomalacia sufferers ultimately may have trouble making it up a flight of stairs and, in the worst cases, might not be able to walk.

The link between vitamin D deficiency and osteoporosis is not as clear. Osteoporosis patients are believed to suffer a calcium deficiency. Some patients do absorb calcium more efficiently with the administration of vitamin D in its hormonal form. Research suggests, however, that not all cases of osteoporosis respond as well to increased vitamin D. An estimated 20 million Americans, most of them postmenopausal women, suffer from osteoporosis, believed to be a result of reduced production of estrogen in the body. This condition interferes with the conversion of vitamin D to a hormone, so the bones are deprived of calcium.

Certain illnesses make it hard for some people's bodies to process vitamin D. These include liver, kidney or parathyroid disease, and vitamin D-dependency rickets, a hereditary disorder. Vitamin D along with calcium has been found useful in treating these problems, but in doses well beyond the RDA of 400 units.

Certain anticonvulsant drugs—phenobarbitol and phenytoin, for instance—also can abnormally speed up the breakdown of vitamin D. Supplementation is required to reverse osteomalacia caused by these drugs but, again, in doses that must be medically prescribed.

Nursing mothers and pregnant women also may require additional vitamin D and calcium. However, in these cases, supplements should *not* be taken without a doctor's recommendation.

Children can also suffer vitamin D deficiency, and their bones, too, can turn soft. This condition in young people, characterized by bow legs and pigeon chest, is called rickets.

In the early days of the Industrial Revolution, as soot, smoke and dust rose high into the sky, blocking sunlight, rickets emerged as a serious problem among children. Today, thanks in large part to vitamin D-fortified dairy products, vitamin D deficiency is uncommon among American children.

Of growing concern, however, are recent reports of vitamin D deficiency among senior citizens, even in the midst of America's Sun Belt.

"What we see happening in our society is that people, particularly as they get older, have a tendency to avoid sunlight purposely," says John L. Omdahl, Ph.D., a biochemist, of the University of New Mexico School of Medicine.

All things being equal, says Dr. Omdahl, a 70-year-old man shouldn't need more vitamin D than a man 50 years younger. As a practical matter, though, many older Americans *do* need more vitamin D because their bodies don't make enough to begin with.

Why not?

There are a variety of reasons, Dr. Omdahl explains.

Many older people worry that exposure to sunlight may lead to skin cancer. Or perhaps they just have trouble getting around, so they remain indoors. And in the winter, in particular, they are reluctant to venture outside into the cold.

Contributing to the deficiency is insufficient vitamin D in the diet. Many older people have trouble digesting milk products, says Dr. Omdahl, so they don't consume enough dairy foods to meet nutritional requirements.

It also is believed that as we get older, our bodies become less able to absorb calcium. Likewise, blood levels of vitamin D hormone also diminish.

Particularly telling is a 1982 study of elderly residents in Albuquerque, New Mexico. According to the study, which Dr. Omdahl coauthored, elderly Americans appear to be getting less vitamin D than the RDA of 400 I.U. Sixty percent of the elderly New Mexicans took in less than 100 units a day. Most were not taking vitamin D supplements and they avoided sunlight, which was abundantly available.

Vitamin D deficiency is uncommon in the United States, says Dr. Omdahl. But among the elderly, particularly city dwellers, vitamin D deficiency *does* occur. "What percentage of the elderly that is, we're still trying to determine," says Dr. Omdahl. "But it is something that should be of concern to the general population."

Lower Sun, Lower Vitamin D Intake

In the winter, getting enough vitamin D can be a problem for anyone living in the northern latitudes. One reason is that the sun is lower in the sky. The sun's ultraviolet rays have trouble punching through the atmosphere, which is thicker at that low angle. There are also fewer hours of daylight and more clouds. Too, when it's cold outside, few of us are inspired to take a sun bath. Sitting next to a nice, sunny window doesn't help, either. Glass filters out Sol's ultraviolet rays.

Suppose you live in West Thumb, Wyoming, and it's been snowing there continually since October. Can you still get enough sunshine to meet your needs? Maybe not. "In the winter, in the northern part of the United States, I'd say the chances are you *aren't* going to get enough vitamin D by skin," says Hector DeLuca, Ph.D., chairman of biochemistry at the University of Wisconsin. For the vulnerable elderly, some of whom may get very little sunlight even in the summer, the need for vitamin D can be particularly acute.

Fortunately, the sun is not the only source of vitamin D. There are some simple ways for the elderly—and the rest of us—to get enough vitamin D while we're huddled up next to the radiator, waiting for spring.

We can consume more dairy foods. If you're tallying up international units of vitamin D, a quart of fortified milk holds 400 I.U.

Vitamin D also is abundant in certain oily fish, such as salmon, mackerel and sardines. You'll find 500 I.U. of vitamin D in 3½-ounce helping of salmon and 275 I.U. in the same size serving of mackerel.

Fish-liver oils are extremely rich in vitamin D. There are, for example, 1,200 I.U. of vitamin D in a tablespoon of cod-liver oil.

Other foods do contain vitamin D, including liver, butter, cheese, eggs and beef. Some cereal products also are fortified. However, vitamin D is not plentiful in vegetables.

Be aware that because the body can store excess vitamin D in fat, large doses of vitamin D, taken over time, can cause serious health problems. That's a very unusual problem, but something to keep in mind. When vitamin D dosage hits the *thousands*-of-I.U. level, that's when trouble can begin.

If too much vitamin D in the diet can cause illness, what about sunshine? Can you overdose on vitamin D after a relaxing afternoon on the golf course? Not to worry. At a certain point, your body knows when to turn off the vitamin D tap. It's self-regulating, like a thermostat.

"Sunshine is the way you were meant to get your vitamin D," says Dr. DeLuca. "The amount of vitamin D that can be made in the skin is limited." We can safely get all the vitamin D most of us require in a multivitamin tablet, which Drs. Ober and DeLuca recommend as "insurance."

"Most of these vitamins have 400 units of vitamin D, which is a safe amount. But I really wouldn't want most people going beyond that," says Dr. Ober.

Why 20 Million People Need More Calcium

There are knowledgeable people in the world who are, for lack of a better phrase, slightly bone dumb; people who think milk is for children and that fibula and tibia are Shakespearean characters; people who believe that brittle bones and the "dowager's hump" are inevitable aspects of growing old. Young women shrug off that clinical-sounding word "osteoporosis" as something that afflicts only grandmothers, and young men tune out talk of the bone-degenerating condition because it's a woman's problem.

It is these people, those whose knowledge of bones comes from cutting apart a frozen chicken, who should consider the words of experts like Jon Block, M.D. "Worrying about osteoporosis after it shows up is like closing the barn door after the horse has already gone. We need to take precautions earlier because you can do very little to reverse the condition once it occurs," says Dr. Block, a member of the osteoporosis research program in the University of California at San Francisco's radiology department.

Previously, osteoporosis efforts have concentrated on treating the condition, but today there's more attention paid to prevention. The target audience is young women, preferably in the teen years, and the goal is to make them aware of changes they can make that could help them avoid the crippling bone condition.

Unwelcome Sign of the Times

Osteoporosis was once scarcely recognized because most people didn't live long enough for their bones to deteriorate. As average life expectancy increased, however, doctors noticed that older women broke their wrists more often than older men, which one German surgeon in 1882 blamed on tripping on long skirts. Wiser men have since put fashion aside and learned that menopause's hormonal changes trigger the loss of bone strength. That's because following menopause there is a dramatic decrease in the production of estrogen, a sex hormone that maintains bone strength.

Today the average woman will live to see at least 78 candles on her birthday cake, which means she will also spend more than one-third of her life in the postmenopausal stage, when osteoporosis is a high risk. "More women are getting older and living longer, as are men, so the situation for both sexes stands to get much worse unless something is done," says James A. Nicotero, M.D., director of the osteoporosis diagnostic center at St. Francis Medical Center in Pittsburgh.

Almost 20 million people have some form of osteoporosis, and at least one million people annually break bones that are weakened by osteoporosis. About 50,000 people die each year from complications due to osteoporosis, with many victims incapacitated for life.

Your Mother Didn't Know

How osteoporosis occurs is clearer now than in mother's day. Calcium, a silver-white metal that's a dominant element in bone, is stored in the skeleton. When more is needed to maintain bones, teeth and other bodily functions than is taken in, a calcium deficiency is created. A federal survey shows that up to 50 percent of males between 18 and 34 have diets deficient in calcium, while two-thirds of women between 18 and 74 fail to take in enough calcium each day.

When the reserves are taxed day after day without being adequately restocked, bones become porous and brittle (hence the name "brittle bone disease") and break easily. Vertebrae can collapse and the resulting dowager's hump can cause severe back pain. Once bone weakens it is difficult to rebuild it to its original strength; there's no cure per se and the objective is to keep the deterioration from worsening.

Women have more trouble with calcium than men and lose bone mass faster, which is why osteoporosis is eight times more common in women. There are plenty of physical factors: Because of smaller body size, women generally have less bone mass to start with; bone loss begins at an earlier age; pregnancy and breastfeeding appear to take a heavy toll, since one skeleton supplies calcium for two lives; women are more likely to go on weight-reducing diets that typically are low in calcium; and women live longer than men.

There are also social factors: Women smoke and drink alcohol more than their grandmothers did, and both smoking and drinking have been implicated in calcium loss; soft drinks and fast foods low in calcium are dietary staples; the think-thin mentality keeps many women away from calcium-rich foods; activity appears to stimulate bone development, but many women live sedentary lifestyles.

Losing Your Bones

"Some bone loss is going to occur in men and women, which is a normal part of the aging process," says Robert Recker, M.D., who has conducted bone research at the Creighton University School of Medicine, in Omaha. "But if lifestyle changes are made early and not just when the prospect of osteoporosis looms overhead, then there's a good chance fractures can be avoided."

Bone mass stops developing at age 35 and bones start slowly losing calcium thereafter until menopause occurs at about age 50 and triggers a more drastic calcium drain. "The strength of a woman's bones at age 35 will determine how she handles the high-risk years," says Stanton Cohn, Ph.D., professor of medicine, school of medicine, State University of New York at Stony Brook, and head of the medical physics division of the Brookhaven National Laboratory, Upton, New York. "The years before age 35 are crucial. A woman can increase calcium intake and exercise between ages 35 and 50 and have some impact, but by that time, all she's trying to do is maintain what's already there."

The amount of calcium needed daily depends on several factors. The government's Recommended Daily Allowance is 800 milligrams. Experts generally agree, however, that the calcium RDA should be higher, possibly 1,200 milligrams for teenagers, 1,000 milligrams for women age 20 through menopause, 1,200 milligrams for pregnant women and anywhere from 1,000 to 1,500 milligrams after menopause, depending on whether estrogen is also being taken.

How to get the necessary calcium depends on personal

preference. A glass of low-fat milk contains about 300 milligrams of calcium, so several would meet the RDA. But there are plenty of other sources: low-fat cheeses, yogurt and ice cream; red kidney, lima and soybeans; blackstrap molasses; fruits, such as watermelon, oranges, raisins and strawberries; fish, especially sardines and salmon when they have soft bones that can be eaten; Brazil nuts, almonds and sunflower seeds; and green, leafy vegetables, which is where the cow gets the calcium for milk in the first place.

Enough calcium can be obtained from food alone. A report in the *New England Journal of Medicine* (January 31, 1985) concluded that the calcium intake of hunter-gatherer tribes still roaming the earth and living lifestyles similar to people who lived in preagricultural days is more than 1,500 milligrams a day, which exceeds the current highest suggested daily requirement. They ingest no dairy products, and possess sturdy bones just by eating which they pluck, pull or catch.

Some people have trouble sticking to a balanced diet, and others just don't like dairy products, in which case calcium supplements may be in order. The most widely recommended are calcium-carbonate tablets, which contain almost three times more calcium than other types of supplements (and that means fewer tablets to swallow).

Some people prefer to take their supplements with meals, while others take them at bedtime; both approaches seem to work, although the experts question whether taking large doses at once is wise. "It's probably best to take it slowly throughout the day instead of in a sudden shot all at once. If you overload, there's a chance that a good bit will be lost through body wastes," says Dr. Cohn.

Moderation is the watchword. Megadoses of calcium that exceed 2,000 milligrams a day can in rare cases lead to kidney stones and constipation.

Swallow and Exercise

Swallowing isn't the only activity that's fundamental in osteoporosis prevention. Exercise is stressed, since the evidence suggests that activity strengthens bone mass. In the younger years almost any form of exercise is beneficial, experts say. For the elderly, brisk walking is recommended. Enjoyment is the key, since the activity must become a routine part of everyday life.

Ironically, it appears that too much exercise can lead to an early onset of osteoporosis. "Young women who exercise to extremes and reduce their body fat levels down to 17 to 20 percent seem to trigger hormonal changes that alter their regular menstrual cycle and cause calcium loss," says Henry A. Solomon, M.D., cardiologist at Cornell University Medical College. "This applies to any actively menstruating woman. Most of the cases that have been seen are women in their twenties and thirties."

Debating Drugs

Taking preventive steps today could spare a woman from becoming entangled in the debate over chemical treatments. In the center of the controversy is estrogen. Some physicians commonly prescribe the drug to postmenopausal women, along with progestogen, which is supposed to protect the uterine lining from cancer that could be caused by the estrogen. Others in the medical community say the treatment hasn't been proved safe.

Meanwhile, sodium fluoride has been added to the fracas. This experimental drug has some practitioners anxiously waiting because there is initial evidence that whereas calcium and estrogen only prevent further bone loss in postmenopausal women, sodium fluoride may make bones stronger.

A new diagnostic device may help prevent women from reaching the stage where any of the synthetic bone drugs are needed. In a 15-minute office procedure, the bone densitometer measures mineral content of the wrist bone at two precise locations, which correspond respectively to both the hipbone and spinal column. The densitometer uses only one one-hundredth the radiation of a standard forearm x-ray, and concentrates the radiation in an area of only two inches; an x-ray scatters radiation to other organs, says Dr. Nicotero, whose diagnostic center includes a densitometer.

"Conventional x-rays can't detect osteoporosis until 30 to 40 percent of the bone mass is lost, in which case bone loss is so extensive that fractures may occur. At that stage, estrogen is often prescribed. The beauty of the densitometer is that we can detect as little as a 2 percent change in bone mass, which means we can initiate therapies before too much damage is done," he says. "So this device could decrease the use of estrogen, because a woman wouldn't be given estrogen if she were found to have excellent bone density at the time of her menopause."

The Effects of Simplicity

With all the information that's surfacing, it would seem that avoiding osteoporosis is simply a matter of drinking milk while exercising in the sun. In this case, however, simplicity is confusing.

"One of the big problems is that the issue of calcium and osteoporosis has been blown out of focus," says David Fardon, M.D., a Knoxville, Tennessee, orthopedic surgeon and author of *Osteoporosis, Your Head Start on the Prevention and Treatment of Brittle Bones* (Macmillan, 1985). "We've paid a lot of attention to the fact that there's not enough calcium in the diet, but the situation has been oversimplified. It's not just a calcium-deficiency disease because there are other factors involved. Some people assume that getting extra calcium will automatically shield them from osteoporosis, but it's not that simple."

Robert Heaney, M.D., who has conducted joint research with Dr. Recker at Creighton University School of Medicine, agrees: "If you go out and buy a bottle of calcium supplements without considering the importance of the other factors, you'll realize some benefit. But if you're striving for the maximum results, you must make sure the other pieces of the puzzle are there also."

For example, researchers at the University of Iowa College of Medicine found that calcium intake alone wasn't related to bone density, but bone density was greater when calcium and vitamin D were adequate (*American Journal of Clinical Nutrition,* vol. 41, no. 5, 1985). But be aware that vitamin D supplements, if taken in excess (the RDA is 400 I.U.), can build up to toxic levels.

Other mysteries of osteoporosis are just beginning to

unravel. In a case involving young and middle-aged men, two groups thought to be safe from osteoporosis, researchers at a Veterans Administration hospital in Illinois found extensive bone loss in those who were chronic alcoholics. The finding enhances previous theories about alcohol interfering with the integrity of the bone.

Of all the questions that remain, one may be the hardest to answer: How do you get a teenager to drink enough milk?

"Brittle bones just don't make a profound impression on the public," says Dr. Fardon. "Also, people want results. They want the satisfaction of seeing their efforts work, and it's not as rewarding to change your lifestyle in the hope of preventing a broken hip decades down the road."

The answer? "Instill good habits while they're children, then they won't have to make any drastic changes later in life when they are set in their ways," Dr. Fardon says. "The best place to start is in the womb, so the child has strong bones when born."

Adds Dr. Block, "Women are flocking to get mammograms because they realize there is the likelihood they could get cancer. But this wasn't always the case, and it took time to get the message out. Today you don't find women asking doctors to measure their bone mass, even though there's a good chance they'll develop osteoporosis. Women don't realize that some of these diagnostic techniques exist. Family physicians will have to do a lot of the motivating, and groups like the Osteoporosis Foundation should help get the message out. The awareness will come, but it will take time."

Healing with Food Fiber

We are living, as one nutritional researcher recently put it, in the era of the "fiber fuss."

Not since Sylvester Graham campaigned for the revival of whole wheat bread in the 1830s has there been so much energy and attention focused on the mainly undigestible portion of the foods we eat—the bran of grains, the pulp of fruit, the crunchy cell walls of vegetables and the squishiness of beans. In other words, the fiber.

Nor have food makers ever shown such an interest in adding more fiber to their products. Having watched the surge in popularity of high-fiber breakfast cereals, food makers are eager to fortify other foods with fiber in hopes of appealing to an increasingly fiber-conscious public.

But the question remains: Why all the fuss?

Because, in the maintenance of good health, fiber plays a role that is even larger than hype. As became evident at a recent major scientific conference on fiber-rich foods sponsored by the University of Delaware's Department of Food Science and Human Nutrition, fiber is an antidote for many of the chronic illnesses that plague us today.

Those illnesses range in severity from hemorrhoids to heart disease, and fiber helps prevent them in several ways. It adds bulk to the diet and relieves constipation, it binds to cholesterol and flushes it from the body, and it speeds up the digestion process, minimizing our exposure to potentially harmful waste products in the intestinal tract. Among those illnesses are:

Appendicitis ● The idea that fiber may prevent appendicitis comes as a surprise. Just this year, researchers at the University of Washington reported the results of a survey comparing the diets of 135 children who had had appendectomies and 212 other children. The children in the upper half of fiber intake were found to be *half* as likely to have developed appendicitis as those in the bottom half. According to researcher Noel Weise, M.D., that means "you could possibly cut the incidence of the disease in half by boosting fiber intake" (*American Journal of Public Health,* April, 1985).

These findings applied only to children and teenagers aged 7 to 18. Another, older study has shown a weak but still positive role for fiber in adults (*Journal of Human Nutrition,* volume 34, 1980).

How might fiber be helping? The appendix is a small blind alley leading off the colon. Hard stools, the kind produced by a low-fiber diet, can get stuck in there, creating an infection and causing the appendix to burst. By keeping stools soft and giving them bulk, fiber prevents the conditions that can lead to appendicitis.

Overweight ● Doctors are recommending bulky, high-fiber foods to their overweight patients because fiber fills them up but not out. High-fiber foods, such as apples, satisfy the appetite while adding very few calories to the meal.

In fact, studies have shown that people lose weight when they eat more fiber, even when they don't go out of their way to change their eating habits. In Sweden, for example, researchers asked a group of women weighing between 150 and 250 pounds to add a supplement of guar gum, a water-soluble form of fiber, or wheat bran to their diets twice a day for ten weeks but not to change their diet in any other way. By the study's end, the women had lost an average of about 15 pounds each (*British Journal of Nutrition,* July, 1984).

Hemorrhoids ● Itching, bleeding and pain are some of the unpleasant but all-too-common symptoms of hemorrhoids, which seem to be the curse of the civilized world. It's an undiscriminating affliction—athletes get them, pregnant women get them and so does half of the entire population over age 50.

But fiber can prevent or relieve hemorrhoids. "A lifetime history of a high-fiber diet is the best way to prevent hemorrhoids, and switching to a high-fiber diet is also the best way to treat many types," says Melvin Bubrick, M.D., a surgeon at Park Nicollet Medical Center in Minneapolis.

"People usually feel better within three or four days after starting a high-fiber diet, but it might take them as long as two weeks to adjust. We recommend unprocessed bran and psyllium-based supplements," he says.

Diabetes ● Not long ago, many adult diabetics resigned themselves to a life of chronic obesity and daily insulin injections. But some doctors are now using high-fiber diets to reduce dramatically diabetic patients' weights and their insulin needs.

"Many diabetics don't need insulin. They need a diet program," says James Anderson, M.D., of the University of

Kentucky, who is a recognized pioneer in the field. "With intensive diet therapy, the majority of diabetic patients can go off insulin."

Using a high-fiber, ultra-low-fat diet, Dr. Anderson claims that he has been able to reduce the insulin needs of his patients anywhere from 25 to 100 percent, depending on the type of diabetes.

Fiber works better for some than for others. "The people who go off insulin entirely usually have only a borderline need for insulin," says James Plonk, M.D., an endocrinologist and diabetes specialist at the Charlotte Memorial Medical Center in Charlotte, North Carolina. "These are people who might not have needed insulin if they'd been eating right all along."

Fiber seems to work by slowing down the release of sugar into the bloodstream, thereby preventing a sudden, enormous demand for insulin, the hormone that guides sugar molecules to the cells to be burned for fuel.

Heart Disease ● Morning joggers who have already quit smoking and switched from beef to fish at suppertime can also protect their hearts another way: by increasing their fiber intake. High cholesterol levels are one of the primary causes of heart disease, and certain kinds of fiber, along with exercise and low-fat foods, seem to bring cholesterol levels tumbling down.

Fiber also acts quickly. In a study by Dr. Anderson, volunteers with cholesterol counts in the caution zone—up around 260 milligrams per deciliter—experienced a 20 percent reduction in cholesterol in only 11 days. All they did was add either of two fiber sources—oat bran or beans—to their daily diet. Otherwise they didn't change their diet at all (*American Journal of Clinical Nutrition,* December, 1984).

Pectin, a form of fiber found especially in apples and citrus fruits, might be the best protection of all against cholesterol-related problems. True vegetarians have unusually low cholesterol levels because of the large amounts of pectin in their diets, according to David Kritchevsky, Ph.D., of the Wistar Institute in Philadelphia.

Some researchers say that these fibers capture excess cholesterol in the digestive tract and flush it out of the body before it can be reabsorbed. Others say that fiber selectively raises the level of HDL cholesterol, the "good" kind of cholesterol that is correlated with a decrease in heart disease.

Colon Cancer ● Cancer of the colon is unlike many other cancers in that it can be detected in its early stages. It may even be preventable if the right approach is used early. The National Cancer Institute believes that fiber might be that approach.

"We feel pretty confident that fiber is involved in the prevention of colon cancer," Joseph Cullen, Ph.D., of the NCI's Division of Cancer Prevention and Control, told us. "It appears that people who eat more fiber have more protection against colon cancer."

Colon cancer is thought to be triggered by the presence of carcinogens in the digestive tract. Sometimes the carcinogens are present in foods, and sometimes they're produced by intestinal bacteria. Either way, fiber may empty the colon faster, flushing out the carcinogens before the body can absorb them.

Diverticulosis ● Thousands of Americans over age 50 are walking around with this disease without knowing it. It is possibly due to increased pressure created in the bowel by constipation, causing little pouches to poke through the intestinal wall like bubbles through a punctured tire. These pouches are called diverticula. Usually they go unnoticed.

Not long ago, the treatment for this disorder was a *low-fiber* diet. Now studies show that the reverse might be helpful. In England last year, researchers took 1,800 rats and fed them either white bread, whole wheat bread or bran along with their usual diet. When examined later, the high-fiber rats had the fewest diverticula. From this, the researchers inferred that doubling the fiber intake of Britons could cut the nation's diverticulosis rate in half (*Lancet*, August 4, 1984).

A high-fiber diet may also ease the pain of infected diverticula (*Federation Proceedings*, July, 1981).

Not All Fiber Behaves Alike

If you are interested in raising your fiber intake in order to prevent illness, keep in mind that not all fiber is alike. One type of high fiber might be great for constipation but not help reduce cholesterol at all.

Wheat bran, for instance, is effective in relieving constipation and possibly the diseases related to constipation. The hemi-cellulose in the bran absorbs water, becomes bulky and promotes regularity.

On the other hand, pectin can help lower cholesterol levels but wheat bran may not. Pectin can be found in apples, oranges, cherries, tomatoes, carrots and other produce. It seems to help remove cholesterol from the digestive tract. So can oat bran and legumes such as brown beans and chick-peas.

Pectin and oat bran can also help diabetics control their blood sugar levels. The fiber present in beans of all kinds works as well, says Dr. Plonk.

Don't make the mistake, however, of going overboard with one kind of fiber or another, or of piling on the bran at every meal. Most Americans, it's said, would be wise to merely double their fiber consumption, from an average of 15 grams up to 30 grams a day. And that should come from a varied diet.

"The best line of advice for the average person is to eat a mix of all the different kinds of fiber," says David Klurfeld, Ph.D., assistant professor at the Wistar Institute. "Eat whole grain foods, fruits and vegetables."

Flush Out Your Body Toxins

Most of us don't work in smelters or foundries any more. But even on Park Avenue, toxins can still enter our bodies and cause slow, subtle damage. Some toxins—potentially deadly— can be created inside our bodies by the normal processes of digestion. Toxins can even be created by our minds: not spiritual poisons but the physical kind, and they can eat your heart out.

Consider an average day in the average life. You arise, get the coffee started and head for a morning shower. Afterward, you get dressed, have a bite of breakfast, wash the few dirty dishes and brush your teeth. The world awaits as you head out the front door, pausing on the stoop to take a deep breath of new morning air.

The day is only an hour or two old, yet there's a chance you may have already encountered several potential toxins. The water used several times could possibly contain slight traces of lead, since the pipes in many homes are held together with a solder that contains the metal. If you live with a cigarette smoker, you may have gotten lead from the smoke. That deep breath before heading off to conquer the day may have included some of the lead in the air that comes from automobile tail pipes.

Unbeknownst to you, there's also a slim chance you've had a brush with cadmium, which like lead, is pervasive in the environment. It can be found in the food chain and in drinking water and the air.

But it may be possible to reduce the danger of these metal pollutants by making sure your diet isn't lacking any of the vital nutrients. Scientists have found that bodies deficient in certain vitamins retain more lead and cadmium.

"We've found that getting enough iron and calcium is a good way to reduce lead damage,"says Kathryn R. Mahaffey, Ph.D., a research chemist who, before joining the National Institute for Occupational Safety and Health, spent ten years researching the dietary effects of lead for the Food and Drug Administration. "By getting enough of these nutrients, you can prevent some of the lead from being absorbed through the gastrointestinal tract. Excessive lead absorption produces brain-cell and kidney damage."

In one calcium experiment, Dr. Mahaffey found that rats eating a diet low in the nutrient and exposed to lead had blood lead concentrations four times greater than rats on a normal calcium diet, although both groups ate the same amount of lead.

In another project, she found that rats given water contaminated with 12 parts per million (ppm) lead and fed a low-calcium diet had tissue lead levels similar to rats receiving water with 200 ppm lead plus normal calcium rations (*Nutritional Reviews,* October, 1981).

A Texas researcher has found that thiamine may have similar protective effects. Working with calves, Gerald Bratton, D.V.M., Ph.D., of Texas A&M University, found that those given toxic doses of lead plus thiamine (vitamin B_1) showed no signs of lead poisoning. "Thiamine in some way prevented the deposition of lead in the tissues examined, especially in the kidneys, liver and brain."

In work with rats, Dr. Bratton found that in those given lead and thiamine, lead levels shot up rapidly, but the metal was soon excreted. "The thiamine helped the lead pass through the rats' bodies instead of it being absorbed into the tissues," he says, adding that the rats showed no adverse effects from the lead.

Dr. Mahaffey stresses that although the nutrients are important, eating patterns seem to be just as crucial. "An adult usually absorbs 5 to 15 percent of the lead that's commonly found in food, whereas after fasting as much as 80 percent of the lead may be absorbed. In other words, don't skip meals or have just a cup of coffee for breakfast."

While lead usually accumulates in the bones, cadmium accumulates in the liver and kidneys. But as with lead, preventing deficiencies of certain vitamins may shield the organs. Some of the most promising work shows iron and vitamin C to be beneficial in preventing the absorption of cadmium.

In research with quail, FDA scientists found that feeding the birds iron and vitamin C reduced the amount of cadmium retained in the kidneys, liver and small intestine. While some protective effect was noted in birds that were given iron only, greater benefits were noted when ascorbic acid was coupled with iron. The scientists speculate that vitamin C improves absorption of iron, which fends off cadmium (*Annals of the New York Academy of Sciences,* 1980).

"We've also had good results with zinc and copper," says M.R. Spivey Fox, Ph.D., who has researched dietary cadmium for the FDA's division of nutrition. "It's important to remember that there's no one natural agent that can rid the body of cadmium once it's absorbed, so no one should start taking large amounts of supplements because that could do more harm than good. Very little cadmium makes its way into the human body, and just avoiding nutrient deficiencies can reduce the amount that's absorbed."

Vitamin B complex may help usher cadmium through the body. Researchers who exposed rats to cadmium and cadmium plus B-complex vitamins found smaller traces of the metal in those animals that received the nutrient. The scientists conclude that one or more constituents of vitamin B complex interfere with the way cadmium normally enters the system and help carry the metal out of the body (*Annals of Clinical and Laboratory Science,* November-December, 1984).

As you move through your day there's a good chance you'll have more than one opportunity to get angry—a chance encounter with an infuriating person, a fender bender in heavy traffic, a slow elevator perhaps. If the rage comes and goes, you're probably okay. But if the feelings persist and you don't vent some steam, a part of your body is physiologically pumping out a potentially toxic substance that's been linked to heart problems and stroke.

The substance is called noradrenaline, and it, along with adrenaline, is triggered into action by the brain when you sense trouble or a threat. These hormones send blood rushing to the muscles, preparing you for swift action (commonly known as the fight-or-flight response). A problem arises when you stay angry and don't vent the hostility, because the brain keeps triggering noradrenaline, which besides threatening the heart may also hamper the immune system.

"Everyday stressors can cause the release of this hormone," says Redford Williams, M.D., an internist who's studied the hazards of hostility, at Duke University Medical Center in Durham, North Carolina. "In lab experiments, we've found that noradrenaline can be released when people are given a difficult math problem to solve. It's very easy to discharge, especially in today's society where there are so many potential irritants."

It's also easy to deal with. "If you blow up and vent your feelings, then you're releasing your anger and in most cases, everything inside will go back to normal and the hormonal release will stop," says Dr. Williams. "Any physical expression that uses up calories, such as exercise, burns up the hormones instead of allowing them to get to the stage in the body where they can do harm. In this case, physical exercise is actually relaxing."

Cholesterol Cops in Action

So now that you've made it through a good portion of the day, it's mealtime. Your daily repasts give you yet another opportunity to do something about substances that can be toxic to your system, such as cholesterol.

You can't see or taste it, but cholesterol is in all foods of animal origin. Some is necessary for proper body function, but you don't need to consume cholesterol—your body will manufacture enough to get by. Like a fat, it won't mix with water, and the body wraps cholesterol in protein packages that help it move through the bloodstream.

One type of cholesterol, known as the HDL variety, causes no harm, whereas the LDL type can be deadly. Too much LDL cholesterol is one of the potentially controllable risk factors for coronary heart disease because it and fats that are also circulating in the blood are deposited on the inner walls of arteries. This narrows the arteries and a blood clot can form at a site of narrowing, which can lead to a heart attack.

Studies have shown you can reduce LDL cholesterol in your blood through dietary means, with fiber from fruits, legumes and vegetables being good vehicles.

Scientists from the Veterans Administration Medical Center and the University of Kentucky in Louisville found that oat bran and beans decreased LDL cholesterol concentrations in men an average of 23 percent. More than two years later, those men who stayed on the high-fiber diet showed a 29 percent decrease in LDL cholesterol levels compared to when they began the study (*American Journal of Clinical Nutrition,* December, 1984).

Fish is another means of reducing cholesterol. The oil in some species of fish—usually those that live in cold climates, such as salmon, tuna, herring, sardines, even lobster and oysters—contains what are known as omega-3 fatty acids, which have been shown to lower levels of LDL cholesterol.

When scientists at Oregon Health Sciences University in Portland fed healthy volunteers diets that included these beneficial fatty acids, LDL cholesterol concentrations fell an average of 20 percent.

If you plan your meals with cholesterol and fat in mind, you may also be taking another positive step toward eliminating an additional troublemaker from your system—bile acids. When fat and cholesterol reach the liver and are metabolized, bile acids are often the by-product. While these acids themselves don't cause cancer, they pave the way for a variety of other factors to come into play, which can lead to colon cancer.

"Some forms of cereal fiber, especially wheat bran, dilute these acids and interfere with their natural functions that can lead to cancer," says Bandaru S. Reddy, Ph.D., who has conducted long-term dietary-fiber research at the Naylor Dana Institute for Disease Prevention, American Health Foundation, Valhalla, New York. "The fiber in the wheat bran increases stool bulk, dilutes the bile acids and binds other tumor-promoting compounds, which are then excreted out of the colon."

In an experiment with rats, Dr. Reddy found that not only did wheat bran protect against colon cancer, but tumors that developed in the animals eating wheat bran were half the size of those found in rats not dining on the fiber.

"Apparently the wheat bran hinders tumor growth. In humans, we could infer that if you eat a diet that includes wheat bran but still develop a colon tumor, there's a chance it may grow at a slower than normal rate. With regular checkups, the tumor would probably be detected, and would be easier to remove with better chances of total recovery," says Dr. Reddy.

What Is a Good Multiple Vitamin-Mineral Formula?

Have you ever stared at a store shelf full of vitamin bottles, totally bewildered? With visions of brightly colored pills spinning through your head, you might well wish for an easier way. Could a multiple vitamin-mineral be just the thing you need?

A multiple combines many nutrients into one tablet or capsule. It's for people who don't want to take five or six, or more, different vitamin pills each day. If it falls short here or there (you may have some special needs), it's easy enough to supplement with additional individual nutrients.

Choosing the multivitamin that's best for you requires a bit of comparison shopping. You need to know how vitamin and mineral supplements meet, or miss, your particular nutrient needs. Here's a step-by-step guide.

One of the best things you can do is compare the list of nutrients on a vitamin bottle label with those in the U.S. Recommended Daily Allowances. Take the table on page 47 with you to the store. Match the label with the table, item for item. Does the multiple include all vitamins and minerals found on the U.S. RDA portion of this table? It should. These are the basics of good nutrition.

Some essential nutrients, especially trace elements, do not yet have U.S. RDAs. They do have safe and accepted ranges, also listed in the chart.

How many of these nutrients are in the multiple? You may not feel you need every one, but you should know which you want, and why. You may want chromium if you're concerned about diabetes (since chromium seems to play a role in glucose metabolism); selenium, a potent antioxidant, because of its possible role in cancer protection; copper if you're taking supplemental zinc. (Copper is important in red-blood-cell formation and capillary stability. Zinc may affect copper absorption. Look for a ratio of about 7.5 to 10 units of zinc to 1 portion copper. For example, 15 milligrams zinc should be taken with 2 milligrams copper.)

There are many other ingredients sometimes found in multiple vitamins—from bioflavonoids to tin. While it's true that these substances are found naturally in food, research has not determined any of them to be essential to human nutrition, at least not yet. If you're looking to get nutritional extras for a special purpose, that's best accomplished through proper food choice or additional supplementation.

Decide How Much You Need

You also should look at the amount of each nutrient in the supplement, listed as milligrams, micrograms (1/1000 of a milligram) or international units (I.U.). Compare each with the U.S. RDA amounts. In addition to amounts, most labels list a nutrient's percentage of the U.S. RDA, and this may actually provide you with the best information regarding the product's potency and balance, as you'll see below.

How potent a multiple do you want? If your goal is "insurance," look for those providing 50 to 150 percent of the U.S. RDA. The American Medical Association considers this a reasonable range. However, the AMA cautions that the vitamin D level should not exceed 100 percent.

Some, but certainly not all, "one-tablet-daily" types are in this category. If you want more than the U.S. RDA, "high-potency" brands may provide it. But so will some other multiples without these labels, says Sheldon Hendler, M.D., Ph.D., clinical instructor of medicine at the University of California at San Diego, and author of *The Complete Guide to Anti-Aging Nutrients* (Simon and Schuster, 1985).

Check for Balance

Look at the percentage of the U.S. RDA of each nutrient. If the formula is balanced by RDA standards, each nutrient will have the same percentage, or multiple, of the U.S. RDA. They'll say "100 percent of U.S. RDA," for instance. If it's not balanced, some percentages will be high, some low.

If the formula doesn't follow the U.S. RDA balance, it's not necessarily bad. But you should note how it varies, and decide if that's something you want.

Some "women's formulas," for instance, contain additional iron or calcium. Some "geri," or geriatric, formulas have additional antioxidants—A, E, C and selenium.

Most of the so-called stress formulas provide much more vitamin C, B complex and, sometimes, zinc than they do other nutrients. Other formulas, like B-100 types, provide equal amounts of all their nutrients. As a result, the formulas may be far out of balance since the U.S. RDAs for some B vitamins are less than one-tenth that of other B vitamins.

"I personally think these products play on the fact that people don't know what 'balanced' is," says Annette Dickinson, technical counselor of the Council for Responsible Nutrition, a vitamin manufacturer's trade association. "It makes no sense to have some of the B vitamins present at 100 times the U.S. RDA, others at only a fraction of the U.S. RDA."

Beware of Supplements That Make Claims

There are now supplement formulas for almost every medical condition you can imagine—arthritis, high blood pressure, heart disease, immunity, depression, fatigue, PMS.

"Be extremely wary of any formula that claims to counteract any particular disease," Dr. Hendler says. "Most of the special formulas I've surveyed are very poorly designed. I think you're better off sticking with a good basic regimen."

But, with your doctor's advice, you may want to take additional vitamins or minerals for a medical problem. If you're a woman, you may take additional iron for anemia, or additional calcium to prevent osteoporosis.

If you have a leg cramping condition called intermittent claudication, your doctor might suggest extra vitamin E. Or he may prescribe B6 and magnesium to help prevent kidney stones, or larger than normal amounts of vitamin C for bronchial asthma. In this sense, the vitamins are going beyond the role of nutrition. They are acting almost as drugs, in a therapeutic sense. Their advantage is that they often have fewer side effects than drugs used for these same conditions. But they still need to be used wisely and under a doctor's supervision. And typically, multiples are not the best way, because the target nutrient is mixed with many others.

Look for the Deficiencies

Some vitamin manufacturers add inadequate amounts of nutrients to their products just so they can list the nutrient on their label, Dr. Hendler says. And even the better products sometimes contain only small amounts of some nutrients. Here again, it's important to read the label.

The once-daily multiple vitamin-mineral supplements are often low in calcium and magnesium, because these two nutrients are bulky and make the pill big. There are many individual calcium supplements on the market these days, though, and some good calcium-magnesium products, which provide

WHAT TO LOOK FOR
IN A FORMULA (U.S. RDA)

Nutrient	Adults and Children 4 or More Years of Age	
Vitamin A	5,000	I.U.
Thiamine (vitamin B_1)	1.5	mg.
Riboflavin (vitamin B_2)	1.7	mg.
Niacin	20	mg.
Vitamin B_6	2	mg.
Folic acid (folacin)	0.4	mg.
Vitamin B_{12}	6	mcg.
Biotin	300	mcg.
Pantothenic acid	10	mg.
Vitamin C (ascorbic acid)	60	mg.
Vitamin D	400	I.U.
Vitamin E	30	I.U.
Calcium	1,000	mg.
Iron	18	mg.
Magnesium	400	mg.
Zinc	15	mg.
Phosphorus	1	gram
Iodine	150	mcg.
Copper	2	mg.
Selenium*,†	50-200	mcg.
Chromium*,	50-200	mcg.

*These nutrients are considered essential, but they have no U.S. RDA. Instead, they have ranges considered safe and adequate.
†Supplements of selenium should not exceed 200 mcg., since the average diet supplies about 100 mcg.

what some researchers think is an important 2.5 to 1 balance between these two minerals. (Magnesium is an important mineral for calcium metabolism.) If you are taking calcium to prevent or treat osteoporosis, you should know some researchers think trace minerals, such as zinc and copper, are very important for bones, too.

Many, but not all, vitamin manufacturers now include an expiration date on their products. It's a good idea to avoid a product beyond that date, although most products retain their potency much longer. Oil-based supplements age more quickly than others. Especially if you're doing your shopping in the store's discount bin, check to see that the vitamins aren't leftovers from the Stone Age.

How Much Can You Swallow?

Some manufacturers that cram everything into a once-daily tablet do so at the expense of your esophagus. Check the pill size before you buy. Sometimes the better choice is to get a just-as-complete, but smaller sized, multiple that must be taken not once, but two or three times a day.

More Is Not Better

You may be tempted to think that if your multiple at its suggested dosage isn't good enough, you can just take it more often and not bother to switch to some better balanced product. You may want more calcium, for instance, but need to take three pills, rather than one, a day. "Don't do that," Dr. Hendler emphasizes. "Taking an unbalanced supplement three times a day still does not provide the recommended doses of some nutrients, but you may end up taking too much of other nutrients, throwing things even further out of balance."

You can do some comparison shopping before you go to the store by looking through the *Handbook of Nonprescription Drugs,* published by the American Pharmaceutical Association, Washington, DC 20037. This book contains a table of many multiple-vitamin products, their ingredients and amounts. The table is a good way to do some comparison shopping before you buy vitamins. The book also includes an RDA chart. Look in the reference section of your library.

Vitamin C Health and Healing Update

● Eighty women seeking Pap smears at the Bronx Municipal Hospital Center may have helped medical science narrow down one of the causes of cervical cancer.

● At a medical research institution in Philadelphia, a labora-

tory experiment turned up unexpected results that may some-day lead to much-needed relief for rheumatoid arthritis sufferers.
● From 1964 to 1978, consumption of vegetables and fruits high in a particular nutrient increased. At the same time, cardiovascular deaths declined. And at least one medical researcher thinks it was no coincidence.

The surprising common denominator, in all cases, is vitamin C.

Although you may have considered vitamin C, or ascorbic acid, essential to everyday good health, a growing body of medical evidence suggests this versatile nutrient may play a more important role in the prevention of disease. Much of this new information is still in the theoretical stage, but it is intriguing.

Here's a wrap-up of recent developments.

Cervical Dysplasia

A low dietary intake of vitamin C is related to cervical abnormalities. That's what Seymour Romney, M.D., found when he tallied up the results of tests comparing women with normal Pap smears and those with cervical cancer or dysplasia—abnormal cell growth that may or may not lead to cancer.

Of the 80 women at the Bronx Municipal Hospital Center who had Pap smears taken, 34 had normal results. Their dietary intake of vitamin C was relatively high. The remaining 46 women took in considerably less vitamin C in the diet, and their diagnoses ranged from mild cervical inflammation to cancer (*American Journal of Obstetrics and Gynecology,* April, 1985).

Just a coincidence—or a connection?

While there's still a lot of work to be done, Dr. Romney believes there is a definite relationship between cervical cancer and low vitamin C in the diet.

"A lot of people have been intrigued by the prospect that vitamin C may have antitumor properties, and there are reasonable scientific studies that support that idea," explains Dr. Romney.

However, how and why vitamin C may prevent tumors from forming isn't well understood. In fact, says Dr. Romney, vitamin C probably is just one part of the picture.

"Cancer is a terribly complicated disease," he says. "With regard to the role of any nutrients, their actions surely involve interactions with other chemicals in the body, which need to be looked into. It's not likely that a single nutrient, per se, is the cause and effect of a disease as complex as cancer."

The preliminary research suggests that women may not be getting enough vitamin C to prevent cervical cancer. Why? Because, says Dr. Romney, "If there's a disorder in the cervix, that increases the demand for ascorbic acid."

Whether you need more than the Recommended Dietary Allowance of 60 milligrams of C daily just isn't clear. However, Dr. Romney and his research staff are attempting to find out. "We're going to try to get some solid information on dosage and the effects of that dosage, whether there are side effects and how well it works."

Of course, cervical cancer is just one of many cancers, and research continues to determine how vitamin C affects them, too.

You might have heard about the link between vitamin C and nitrosamines, cancer-causing substances formed by the interaction of nitrites—a common food additive—and chemicals in your body.

Vitamin C has long been believed to prevent nitrosamines from forming. A recent study reported in the journal *Carcinogenesis* (vol. 6, no. 11, 1985) lends strong support to that theory.

Researchers in Britain asked eight volunteers to take a gram (1,000 milligrams) of vitamin C every day for a week. Before and after the experiment, researchers siphoned off gastric juice from the volunteers' stomachs. In all but one of the volunteers, levels of nitrosamines in the gastric juice were significantly lower at the end of the test.

Does this mean vitamin C prevents gastric cancer? No, but it may reduce the risk. Are the results definitive—that is, is this the last word? No. Further studies, and on a wider scale, should be done before coming to any definite conclusions. But the results of this study do give reason for optimism.

Picture the body at war with itself. That's what happens in rheumatoid arthritis. The body's own cells mistake body tissues for foreign substances. To repel the "invaders," the cells manufacture antibodies to attack the tissue.

There is no cure for rheumatoid arthritis. Treatment often involves using steroids to reduce the pain and tissue swelling brought about by this disfiguring disease. But these anti-inflammatory drugs in themselves can cause side effects.

That's why Robert H. Davis, Ph.D., a professor in the department of physiology at the Pennsylvania College of Podiatric Medicine, has been exploring the use of vitamin C and aloe, two natural substances that cause no side effects.

"It's an idea that goes back, for me, almost 30 years," says Dr. Davis. "Steroids and synthetic drugs have their place in the treatment of arthritis, but the side effects can sometimes be worse than the cure."

Why vitamin C? Simply this, says Dr. Davis: Vitamin C is an essential building block in the manufacture of the connective tissue called collagen. In rheumatoid arthritis, this connective tissue breaks down. But Dr. Davis believes that vitamin C, applied to the skin, may prevent or slow this tissue breakdown, reducing inflammation. And aloe also is believed to have healing properties.

In a prize-winning study that put his theory to the test, Dr. Davis and two students combined vitamin C, aloe and ribonucleic acid—a cellular building block also thought to reduce inflammation—in a cream ointment. Then they applied the cream to the arthritic hind paws of laboratory rats. The results were surprising. Joint-tissue swelling was reduced dramatically, both in the early stages of arthritis and later on, after the disease had progressed for several days (*Journal of the American Podiatric Medical Association,* May, 1985).

"I honestly didn't think it would work," said Dr. Davis. "But I was able to repeat the results."

Of course, it is too soon to say what impact these studies will have on humans. Furthermore, it's important to understand that this report is by no means a cure for rheumatoid arthritis. But it offers some hope for an effective treatment that doesn't rely on steroids.

"I wouldn't recommend this kind of treatment to anyone until we get some real statistical data," says Dr. Davis. "I would like to say yes because rheumatoid arthritis is one of the tough ones. But I think it first has to go into a clinical trial and be evaluated. If somebody has a real bad case of arthritis, they should be treated by a doctor."

Most animals make their own vitamin C. In fact, there are only a few species—humans, guinea pigs, monkeys and certain fruit bats—that have to get their vitamin C from what they eat.

Members of the one civilized, self-aware species in that group appear to suffer a chronic dietary shortage of vitamin C, says Anthony Verlangieri, Ph.D., of the University of Mississippi. And because of that deficiency, he says, "they may be more susceptible to heart disease."

Dr. Verlangieri believes vitamin C deficiency causes atherosclerosis. True, cholesterol does clog arteries. But in Dr. Verlangieri's view, cholesterol is really a Johnny-come-lately, a cardiovascular bad guy who takes advantage of an already bad situation caused by a vitamin C deficiency.

One recent study by Dr. Verlangieri and colleagues at the University of Mississippi lends support to his theory.

Dr. Verlangieri and his staff reviewed health statistics ranging from 1964 to 1978. During that time, he noticed, Americans increased their intake of fruits and vegetables rich in vitamin C. Deaths from cardiovascular disease during that period declined.

Other experts also have noted the decline in cardiovascular deaths and have attributed the slide to a number of factors, including a reduction in smoking, better eating habits and an increase in physical activity.

But in his study, Dr. Verlangieri credited the increased intake of foods rich in vitamin C for the decline in heart deaths (*Medical Hypotheses,* volume 16, 1985).

According to Dr. Verlangieri's research, vitamin C turns off an enzyme that attacks the cells—endothelial cells, they are called—in blood-vessel walls. If you are vitamin C deficient—that is, if your cells aren't saturated with vitamin C—the enzyme is free to do its dirty work.

"The cells of blood vessels can be compared to bricks in a wall," explains Dr. Verlangieri. "Mortar holds the bricks in the wall together, but in blood vessels, a cement called the extracellular matrix holds the cells together. If the cement becomes defective, the cells loosen up. That leaves some bare spots. Normally, the cells provide a barrier to keep cholesterol off the blood-vessel walls. But when the cholesterol gets into those bare spots, it causes inflammation. Vitamin C actually works at the level of the cell to inhibit an enzyme that chews up that cement."

If the body is low in vitamin C, the blood-vessel walls become denuded in spots, says Dr. Verlangieri, leaving convenient places for cholesterol to take root. So cholesterol is an important part of the process once the disease begins, but it isn't how the disease begins.

How much vitamin C, then, do people need to prevent cardiovascular disease? According to Dr. Verlangieri, the RDA of 60 milligrams isn't enough. "I think the evidence suggests that from 1,000 to 2,000 milligrams is probably what we need," he says.

Before you consider increasing your intake of C, bear in mind that in many quarters this theory is still controversial. Some scientists do not think vitamin C is involved in coronary artery disease. Others do believe vitamin C appears to reduce coronary risks, but for altogether different reasons.

For instance, one study suggests vitamin C in 1,000-milligram doses prevents blood platelets from clumping together and adhering to blood-vessel walls. To find out whether this is true, researchers at Tagore Medical College and Hospital in India gave volunteers 1,000 milligrams of vitamin C every eight hours for ten days. At the end of that period, they drew blood samples and found a significant drop in the rate at which blood platelets clumped together and adhered.

But at the same time, the research scientists noted that they were administering vitamin C in "pharmacologic doses" —doses so high they should be taken only under a doctor's supervision. They concluded that further studies needed to be done to confirm their findings (*Clinical Cardiology,* vol. 8, no. 10, 1985).

Whatever the connection, recent research at least suggests that there might be one. And that meets with Dr. Verlangieri's approval. "Most animals produce their own vitamin C, sometimes from 5 to 20 grams a day," he says. "There must be a reason why they make so much. That's why I believe the RDA is very, very low. The RDA also does not take into account factors such as lifestyle, medications and smoking that deplete the body's levels of vitamin C. Sixty milligrams a day is just too low to keep you at a saturated level."

FOOD SOURCES OF VITAMIN C

Food	Portion	Vitamin C (milligrams)
Orange juice, fresh	1 cup	124
Grapefruit juice, fresh	1 cup	94
Papayas	½ medium	94
Strawberries, sliced	1 cup	85
Kiwi fruit	1 medium	75
Oranges	1 medium	70
Green peppers, raw, chopped	½ cup	64
Mangoes	1 medium	57
Cantaloupe	¼ medium	56
Cranberry juice cocktail	½ cup	54
Brussels sprouts, cooked	4 sprouts	52
Tomato juice	1 cup	45
Grapefruit, white	½ medium	44
Broccoli, raw, chopped	½ cup	41
Kale, raw chopped	½ cup	41
Cauliflower, raw, chopped	½ cup	36
Potatoes, baked	1 medium	26
Tangerines	1 medium	26
Tomatoes, raw	1 medium	22
Turnip greens, cooked	½ cup	20
Dandelion greens, raw, chopped	1 cup	19
Beet greens, cooked	½ cup	18
Cabbage, raw, shredded	½ cup	17

SOURCES: *Composition of Foods: Fruits and Fruit Juices,* Agriculture Handbook No. 8-9, and *Composition of Foods: Vegetables and Vegetable Products,* Agriculture Handbook No. 8-11, U.S. Department of Agriculture.

Men Only/Women Only Nutrition Guidance

He may say tow-may-tow, and she may say tow-mah-tow, but who's more likely to eat it and benefit from its potassium, vitamins A and C, fiber, low calories and low fat? She is. Chances are he'll get his tow-may-tow as a smear of ketchup on a hamburger.

Studies show that men and women eat differently, and that they have distinct nutritional needs.

Food preference surveys, for instance, show that men are nearly twice as likely as women to eat whatever they want, and that what they want is a high-fat cut of red meat. That's one reason that, even in these health-conscious times, the typical man's diet is too high in fat, and sometimes low in the vitamins and minerals found in fruits, vegetables and dairy products.

Women like meat, too, but they also want fruits and vegetables. Their food shopping and cooking skills make them likely to be more nutritionally aware than men, but they also have special dietary demands, particularly during pregnancy. And they're twice as likely as men to be watching their weight, possibly eating too few calories to supply all the nourishment they need, especially during their childbearing years.

The National Academy of Sciences' Recommended Dietary Allowances reflect most, but not all, of the differences in nutritional requirements between the sexes. At every age men require 10 to 30 percent more protein, vitamins A, E, thiamine, riboflavin, niacin and B_6, and magnesium than women. They require equal amounts of vitamins D, C, folate and B_{12}, calcium, phosphorus, zinc and iodine. They require only about half as much iron.

Women who are pregnant or breastfeeding an infant have the highest nutritional requirements. They need as many or more vitamins and minerals as men. In some cases—with folate and calcium, for instance—their needs jump dramatically. Not meeting those needs can result in low-birth-weight babies or seriously impair the mother's health.

55

Iron Requirements

Iron is one nutrient women need more of than men, according to the National Academy of Sciences. Menstruating women require almost twice as much iron as men (18 milligrams compared to men's 10 milligrams). And pregnant women may need 30 to 60 milligrams of iron each day.

Nutritional surveys show that about 40 percent of women of childbearing age don't get enough iron, says Cecilia Davis, a registered dietitian who directs a nationwide dietitian's referral service, the Consulting Nutritionist Practice Group.

"Women absorb only about 6 milligrams of iron per 1,000 calories of food in a typical diet," she says. "They would need to eat about 3,000 calories a day to meet their iron RDA. Few eat that much, so many women need supplemental iron."

Teenage girls are even worse off, Davis contends. "I'd say 80 percent could be iron deficient. Some eat as few as 1,000 calories a day, and their food preferences are poor in iron."

Among teenagers, boys can also develop iron deficiencies, sometimes rather quickly when they start the rapid growth of adolescence. There is an enormous demand for blood-building materials at this stage. "And I'd say this is more likely to be overlooked in boys than in girls," Davis says.

Both adult men and women may sometimes become iron depleted during very strenuous athletic training, says Paul Zabetakis, M.D., a research physician at the Institute of Sportsmedicine and Athletic Trauma in New York. In super-athletes, pounding exercise can actually break down red blood cells and lead to anemia (iron deficiency).

Dr. Zabetakis cautions that average runners (as well as ultramarathon athletes) may also develop "pseudo-anemia." Blood tests will show lower-than-normal iron levels, but the larger volume of blood they have developed as a result of their athletic activities means their oxygen-carrying capacity remains the same. They'll have no physical symptoms of anemia.

When most adult men (and women past menopause) develop iron deficiencies, though, it's usually not exercise or diet that's at fault, says Robert McGandy, M.D., a Tufts University professor of medicine and consulting doctor for the

Boston-based Human Nutrition Research Center for Aging. Internal bleeding—ulcers, intestinal polyps, excessive aspirin or alcohol use, even hemorrhoids—are too often the cause. "In this case, it's important to be checked for blood loss, and not to try to cure yourself with an iron supplement," Dr. McGandy says.

Everyone, but especially men, small children and post-menopausal women, can develop iron overload. They can take in so much iron that it builds up in their liver or spleen and begins to cause damage. (It can also make it difficult to travel by air. One man with this problem found it impossible to get by the metal detector at an airport. He'd been getting frequent blood transfusions for a medical problem.)

"Nobody is going to get an overload, though, unless he's getting at least five to ten times the RDA," Dr. McGandy says. "No man is going to get this just by taking his wife's multivitamin with iron."

Mother's Helper

Sometimes what masquerades as an iron deficiency is actually a folate problem. One common nutritional problem in the United States is a low intake of this B vitamin. People just aren't eating enough folate-rich dark green leafy vegetables, and women, especially, pay the consequences.

Anemia can occur when there is not enough folate in the body to produce red blood cells. Among older women, especially, folate, rather than iron, may be the culprit in this problem. And folate deficiencies have been implicated in cervical dysplasia, a condition that can lead to cancer of the cervix. The vitamin has also been found to reverse the disease in some women.

Pregnant women need to double their folate intake from 400 to 800 micrograms, and those who are breastfeeding need 500 micrograms. "Folate is needed for the manufacture of all cells," Dr. McGandy says. That's why it's so important to fetal growth and growth of the newborn baby. In fact, both spina bifida, a birth defect in which the tissue around the spinal cord doesn't close properly, and cleft palates have been associated with low folate intake. In one study, women who had had one baby with spina bifida were much less likely to have a second baby with the same problem if they got adequate folate.

Vitamin B_6 has been associated with "women's problems" for some time now. It's been used to treat fluid retention and other symptoms associated with premenstrual syndrome. It's also been prescribed for women taking birth-control pills, who often have lower blood levels of this vitamin. Mood changes, like depression, that some women taking birth-control pills experience, have been attributed to lower levels of B_6, which some researchers speculate may lead to decreased production of the brain neurotransmitter serotonin. See your doctor if you think you need more than 25 milligrams a day of B_6. High doses have been associated with neurological changes.

The Discriminating Mineral

The RDA chart lists the same calcium requirement, 800 milligrams a day, for men and women. This does not reflect the growing belief among nutritionists that women need more than this amount to prevent osteoporosis. Some feel that younger women need 1,000 milligrams and postmenopausal women up to 1,500 milligrams a day of calcium to help prevent this crippling disease of older women.

The problem is that many women don't even get 800 milligrams a day, Davis says. Calcium deficiencies among women are second only to iron. The average intake for women is 600 milligrams.

"Getting 1,000 milligrams a day of calcium means three or four servings of high-calcium foods, mostly dairy products," Davis says. "Although you can get this amount of calcium through foods—and that's the best way—it does take quite a bit of attention to do so without taking in a lot of calories." Low-fat dairy products or calcium supplements provide bone-building material without the fat-building side effects.

You might think scurvy had disappeared along with pirates and wooden galleons, but that's not what some doctors have found.

It's true that in these days of year-round fresh fruit and instant breakfast juices scurvy is uncommon in the United States. Just about everyone gets at least the 10 milligrams of vitamin C needed to ward off this disease.

But not everyone does, as doctors at the Veterans Administration Medical Center in Portland, Oregon, recently discovered. Each of the three men they saw had swelling, pain and purplish bruising of their legs, along with other symptoms like gum disease, fatigue, blood in the stools or, the classic scurvy tipoff, corkscrew hair. Two had undergone extensive medical testing to try to determine the cause of their symptoms.

But it was an analysis of their diet, and a check of their blood levels of vitamin C, that led to correct diagnosis—scurvy. It turned out all three lived alone, cooked for themselves or ate out. Each admitted he rarely ate fresh fruits or vegetables. Supplemental vitamin C eliminated their symptoms in just a few days (*Journal of the American Medical Association,* February 8, 1985).

Because scurvy is rare, physicians may not recognize it when they see it, the Portland doctors say. Men who live alone and cook for themselves, especially the elderly or heavy drinkers, are among those at highest risk for developing scurvy, they say.

The Fiber Factor

Turning up their noses at fruits and vegetables can have other consequences for men. "We tend to see too little fiber in their diets," says Rebecca McCully, R.D., consulting nutritionist for the Cardiovascular Clinic in Oklahoma City. "Men who have very sedentary jobs and eat low-fiber diets are more likely to develop chronic constipation. Women are less prone to this problem because they tend to eat a lot more fresh fruits and vegetables."

Admittedly, the men she sees may eat less well than some—after all, they've had heart problems. "The biggest problems I see in people's diets are excesses—too much fat, salt, calories," she says. Nutritional deficiencies are much less common, at least in the middle-class Midwestern men she sees. In any case, her advice applies equally well to men and women.

"I tell my people that their doctors aren't responsible and their spouses aren't responsible for what they put in their mouths. They are, and they must accept that responsibility and learn to make healthy food choices and decisions."

"Feel-Better" Foods

You feel hot, but shivers run though your aching muscles. Your stuffy head feels like it's wearing a steel helmet several sizes too small. You squint at the column of mercury in the thermometer—hovering around 101 degrees.

Face it. You've got what six fellow workers have come down with—the flu.

Now you're in a quandary. Your mother always told you to starve a fever and feed a cold. What do you do now that you have both?

If you respond to your growling stomach, will your fever run riot? If, on the other hand, you fail to feed that cold, will it find more organs in your body to torment?

"The best advice is to forget that old bromide," says Jay Swedberg, M.D., assistant professor of family practice, University of Wyoming, "and let your appetite be your guide."

If the heady fumes from the kitchen make you hungry, by all means indulge it with small, infrequent snacks, Dr. Swedberg advises. "Your feverish body needs nutrients to keep up your strength and your spirits."

That's because fever, while stoking your body's defense machinery, also speeds up your metabolism, which raises your requirements for liquids, protein, calories and all other nutrients.

Ironically, even though your nutrition needs are soaring, your appetite tends to plummet. Mocha layer cake has no charms, and even sick children frequently go on a closed-mouth strike that their most favorite foods will not pry open.

What do you eat if you're not hungry? "Nothing," says

Mike Oppenheim, M.D., a Los Angeles physician board certified in family practice. "It's common to lose your appetite during an illness, especially the flu.

"Many people think that lack of food will slow their recovery." Not so, says Dr. Oppenheim. "The average adult has ample reserves of protein, fat and other nutrients."

In fact, lack of appetite might be body wisdom in action. There is some evidence that withholding nourishment is the body's attempt to starve the microorganisms that are causing the infection.

"But you must have fluids," Dr. Oppenheim cautions. "In order to cool you down, your fever causes you to perspire. Unless the lost fluid is replaced you may become dehydrated. Your body will protect itself from further water loss by cutting down on sweating, making it more difficult for you to cope with fever.

"If your temperature is no higher than 101 for a day or two, dehydration is not a real threat. But if you have the flu with higher fevers that fluctuate up and down for a week, your fluid intake is critically important," Dr. Oppenheim told us. "If you're an adult with a high fever, your body may need two extra quarts of water a day. If you are nauseated, suck on ice or lollipops. You'll probably be urinating a little more than usual. If not, drink more."

"For a routine bout with the flu, take your fluids in small sips," Dr. Swedberg advises. What should you sip? "Try apple juice diluted half-and-half with water. Undiluted fruit juices have too much sugar in this situation. A little sugar provides necessary glucose but excess sugar can cause diarrhea when you're ill. Ginger ale and other nondiet soft drinks should also be diluted with water and allowed to sit until they go flat. Carbonation can create gas in the stomach, which can make you more nauseated."

Ice cubes made from diluted juice with a grape or a strawberry embedded in each may entice a feverish child. So will fruit-flavored gelatin.

"When you're feeling queasy, citrus juices should be avoided," Dr. Swedberg advises. "They tend to aggravate an already upset stomach. If there is vomiting or diarrhea, milk is not advised. Yogurt, however, is fine. It helps to reestablish a healthy microbial environment in the colon."

Yogurt can be whizzed in a processor with a touch of vanilla and a little honey to make a pleasant sipable beverage.

"To make the transition from liquids to more substantial fare, put the emphasis on bland starchy foods," Dr. Swedberg advises. "Dry toast is fine. Try bananas, applesauce, cottage cheese, baked potatoes, which could be topped with yogurt or cottage cheese, boiled rice or rice pudding and cooked cereals." For a refreshing dessert try banana ice dessert made from frozen very ripe bananas whizzed in the food processor.

If, however, lack of appetite persists for five days or you have lost 5 percent of your weight, consult a physician or a registered dietitian. You may need a nutritional formula designed for flagging appetites, advises George Blackburn, M.D., director of nutrition at New England Deaconess Hospital.

After the fever breaks, watch out! Your appetite will return with a vengeance. "Make the most of it," Dr. Blackburn counsels, "until you regain your lost weight, but keep it wholesome. Your ravenous appetite is a response to your body's attempt to replenish nutrients and rebuild tissue destroyed during the infection. Protein and calories are the most important factors in a recovery diet, but make a conscious effort to include foods that also restore the water-soluble vitamins B and C."

Children will gobble up double the calories of their normal diet. "Don't wean children back on a solid diet through the old-fashioned tea-and-toast route," Dr. Blackburn cautions. "Their craving for food is a good sign and should be met with good solid food. If they crave hamburgers and milkshakes, that's fine. If they want steak, lamb chops, mashed potatoes, rejoice. They are on the road to recovery and their bodies are eager to make up for lost nutrients."

Foods That Soothe a Cold

Hot tea with a little honey is a tried-and-true remedy for a stuffy nose. "Inhaling steam loosens mucus in the nasal passages, helping to wash away infecting organisms," says Joseph Vitale, M.D., Sc.D., head of the department of nutritional pathology at Boston University School of Medicine. "But chicken soup works even better. Nobody knows why but no one will deny that steaming chicken soup is balm not only to the body, but makes the spirits soar. And that can speed recovery.

"The warmth and affection with which food is offered has a very strong placebo effect. The message of caring that garnishes the soup and other dishes you take pains with may do more good than the food itself," he adds.

"For a more vigorous effect on your sinuses, try something spicy," suggests Irwin Ziment, M.D., director of respiratory therapy and chief of medicine at Los Angeles County Olive View Medical Center.

"Mexicans living in Los Angeles who go in for hot, spicy foods, even though they suffer exposure to smog, have fewer problems with bronchitis than non-Mexicans who have bland diets," Dr. Ziment notes.

"Use lots of horseradish, mustard, cayenne, chili pepper and garlic on your food," he advises. "Enjoy oysters with horseradish and Tabasco, spiced shrimp cooked Creole-style in Tabasco, highly seasoned gumbo laced with garlic, which is a worldwide recognized expectorant. Such hot, spicy food—by loosening up your abnormal secretions—clears your sinuses, your nose and your lungs."

For those with an ulcer or a stomach intolerant of spicy food, Dr. Ziment has another suggestion: "Sprinkle 20 drops of Tabasco sauce into a glass of water, and gargle but don't swallow.

"For a sore throat, try chewing on cloves. They have an anesthetic quality. Use no more than four a day for adults; children should have no more than three," Dr. Ziment cautions. "And mint tea has a soothing effect on a throat that is raspy. Try it cold initially, then after a day or so, switch to hot drinks with a little honey." Or try Dr. Ziment's favorite Russian remedy—one teaspoon pure horseradish and one teaspoon honey stirred into a glass of warm water. "Sip it slowly, keep stirring as the horseradish tends to settle, and think happy thoughts," he says.

Children and Diarrhea

If a child has an intestinal virus with severe diarrhea, should he eat solid foods, clear liquids or nothing at all? Twenty years ago, pediatricians as a rule advised letting the bowel rest for 24 to 48 hours, then reintroducing foods slowly over the next few days.

Bul William J. Klish, M.D., head of pediatric gastroenterology at Baylor College of Medicine and chief of nutrition and gastroenterology at Texas Children's Hospital, in Houston, advises against this procedure. "A prolonged period of starvation may be dangerous.

"A child who is not dehydrated and can keep food down should be fed a normal diet," Dr. Klish told us.

"Avoid undiluted fruit juices," Dr. Klish advises. "They prolong vomiting and apple juice can promote diarrhea. Yogurt is a good food for these children."

What do you feed a dehydrated child? "If the child is dehydrated, and you can spot this by signs of dry mouth, dry skin and irritability, he should be under the care of a physician, who may prescribe an oral rehydration formula."

What if the child is vomiting? "Bland foods or, for infants, half-strength formula should be given for the first day, and solid foods (bananas, rice cereal, applesauce and toast) begun as soon as the child can tolerate them. Breast-fed infants should continue on the breast. Breast milk is well tolerated and contains helpful antibodies."

What if the diarrhea persists? "Diarrhea that lasts more than two weeks should be investigated for the possibility of lactose intolerance or celiac disease, which is an intolerance to gluten," says Dr. Klish. "The gluten damages the lining of the small intestine, causing malabsorption of foods. Those with this disorder, called sprue in adults, should substitute corn, rice, soy and amaranth, which have no gluten, for gluten-containing wheat and rye."

Nutritional "Boosters" for Your Middle Years

So you've left dissipated youth and its wild excesses behind. You've reached whatever the current generation considers middle age—anywhere from 40 to 60. You're on top of the hill, enjoying the view, and you want to be able to stay there a good long time. You want the second half of your life to be as healthy and active as possible.

Your concerns are shared by scientists exploring the connection between aging and nutrition. These researchers, several of whom presented their work recently at the Bristol-Myers/Tufts University Symposium on Nutrition and Aging, are discovering that many diseases traditionally associated with aging are strongly influenced by other factors, especially poor nutrition. They're looking at the possibility of increased nutrient needs for older adults. And they're seeing that any good nutritional program intended to lighten the load of old age is best started during middle age—before you head down the hill.

It's well known that older people are at higher risk for developing low nutrient levels, even when they're healthy, educated and well off.

One reason for this is simply a matter of numbers, says Walter Mertz, M.D., director of the U.S. Department of Agriculture's Agricultural Research Service, Human Nutrition Research Center in Beltsville, Maryland. "As they age, people eat less and less, until at about age 70 they're getting 20 percent fewer calories than they were at age 40. Their average calorie intake becomes too low to meet the Recommended Dietary Allowance for a number of nutrients." Combine this with less-than-ideal food choices and you're setting the stage for the marginal intakes found among older adults for calcium, B complex, vitamins C and A, zinc, iron, copper, chromium, even protein.

Dr. Mertz is particularly interested in pinpointing the consequences of chronic marginal intakes of trace minerals like zinc, copper, chromium and silicon (an element proved necessary for animals but not humans).

Zinc, copper and silicon, for instance, are important in maintaining bone tissue. Dr. Mertz would like to see if people with osteoporosis are deficient in these trace elements. "We must get away from focusing just on calcium while we ignore other nutrients involved in osteoporosis," he says. "This condition may be the result of multiple deficiencies and requires a total nutritional approach."

While supplements may help, they aren't always the answer, Dr. Mertz says. "The ideal solution would be to increase your activity level as much as you can, to boost your appetite and food intake," he says.

People with osteoporosis may also have osteomalacia, says Michael F. Holick, Ph.D., M.D., director of the Vitamin D and Bone Metabolism Laboratory at the USDA Human Nutrition Research Center on Aging at Tufts University, in Boston.

Osteomalacia is a vitamin D-deficiency disease that keeps bone tissue from mineralizing and becoming hard. It's common in northern Europe, where milk is not fortified with vitamin D. It was thought uncommon in the United States, but that's not what Dr. Holick found when he collaborated in a survey of patients coming into Massachusetts General Hospital with hip fractures. "We found 40 percent were vitamin D deficient, and 30 percent had clear signs of osteomalacia," he says.

Getting this vitamin's RDA of 400 international units is sufficient, Dr. Holick says. That's the amount found in most multivitamin tablets, or in four eight-ounce glasses of fortified milk. Another source of vitamin D is sunlight. (Vitamin D is made in the skin on exposure to sunlight, but this ability decreases with age.) Wearing a sunscreen will block vitamin D production, so Dr. Holick suggests waiting 10 to 30 minutes (but before sunburning occurs) before applying.

But you don't have to trade off osteoporosis for skin cancer, insists Barbara Gilchrest, M.D., chairman of the dermatology department at Boston University's School of Medicine.

Like other organs in the body, the skin's function declines as we age. It becomes dry, wrinkled and takes longer to heal.

But that decline may be more a matter of diet and exposure to sunlight than to passing years, Dr. Gilchrest says.

"Diet and exposure to sun probably cause most of the changes we think of as aging. We know the sun can damage cell membranes and genetic structure and that diet can exert positive or negative effects on the skin."

Dr. Gilchrest discovered one positive nutritional effect using beta-carotene, a form of vitamin A found in yellow, orange and red vegetables. She grew human skin cells in culture, some with and some without beta-carotene. Then, she exposed the cells to increasingly strong amounts of harmful sunlight. At the first two exposures (equivalent to moderate sunburn) the cells receiving the beta-carotene showed significantly fewer signs of damage than the cells without beta-carotene. "They grew normally and looked better," Dr. Gilchrest says. "In fact, they looked just like the control cells, which had received no radiation at all." At the highest level of exposure, the cells did show some damage, but still not as much as those without beta-carotene.

It would be premature to translate this finding into recommendations for people, Dr. Gilchrest says. "Beta-carotene does seem to protect cells from damage, but I can't tell you how many carrots a day you should be eating." At least not yet.

"This type of work allows us the prospect of really knowing in some scientific way what the diet should be," Dr. Gilchrest says. "Up to now it has been a guessing game. The RDAs are based on very coarse kinds of studies, feeding or not feeding animals something and seeing if they get sick. But this type of work allows us to say, 'This is what the food is actually doing for you, and according to these experiments these are the consequences if these levels aren't met.' "

As Goes Skin, So Goes the Body

Skin might provide an easy-to-observe model for testing theories of nutrient protection for other parts of the body, Dr. Gilchrest says. "There's evidence that damage similar to the type sunlight causes to the skin is produced inside the body by some foods, chemicals and everyday metabolic reactions." Exposure to these things can cause the formation of errant molecules called free radicals, which damage body parts just as surely as they rust iron or spoil food. In fact, one "theory" of aging contends that the process is a buildup of free-radical damage to body tissues.

That's probably not the whole story, but it's a place to start, at least when you are looking at possible nutritional intervention, says Jeffrey B. Blumberg, Ph.D., associate professor of nutrition at Tufts and acting associate director at the Human Nutrition Research Center on Aging at Tufts.

"We know that animals deficient in antioxidants like vitamins E, C and A and selenium develop cell damage similar to that seen with aging," Dr. Blumberg says. "But in experiments where animals are given supplemental antioxidants, it's not clearly shown that these nutrients alter the basic aging rate. That is, it's not clear that they extend the maximum life span of the animals, although they do seem to increase the average life span because they reduce the incidence of early death from diseases like cancer."

As pieces of the aging puzzle come together, though, evidence seems to indicate an increased need for certain antioxidants in some tissues. Dr. Blumberg's work so far has focused mostly on the cells of the immune system and their interaction with vitamin E.

With age, the immune system slows, leaving the body more open to infection. Important to the immune response are white blood cells known as lymphocytes. When the body senses a "foreign invader" like a bacterial infection, the lymphocytes proliferate in great numbers, then move in to destroy the bacteria. This process is slower in old than in young animals. But Dr. Blumberg found that old animals given supplemental vitamin E had a significant boost in proliferation and activity of lymphocytes. He's now doing an experiment to see if the same thing happens in humans.

"We are giving 800 I.U. a day of vitamin E to healthy elderly volunteers to see whether the animal results we found are matched in humans. We'll be measuring a number of immune-response parameters, including lymphocyte proliferation," he says.

One thing Dr. Blumberg noticed in his lymphocyte study

were changes in body balance of an important group of biochemicals called prostaglandins. These chemicals influence
many functions in the body, including blood clotting, the
production of neurotransmitters, and the production of the
body's own free-radical "quenchers." The balance of
prostaglandins changes to an apparently less-favorable mix as
we age, and Dr. Blumberg believes this may be an important
mechanism in the development of age-related declines in function. If he's right, it could mean that vitamin E's effect is
pervasive throughout the body and that it could influence a
number of aging-related conditions—kidney failure, cataracts,
atherosclerosis, even some nervous system and brain functions.

He's found, for instance, that the cerebellum and brain
stem have high metabolic needs for vitamin E. Among other
things, these two regions of the brain control reflexes. One of
the first symptoms of vitamin E deficiency is loss of reflex
response. Could older people be losing their reflexes because
of low vitamin E intake? Dr. Blumberg would love to find out.

With further study, there may well be recommendations
for increased intake of antioxidants as we age, Dr. Blumberg
says. "But there's a certain irony in talking about higher doses
when we know that many older people are not getting even the
RDA of these vitamins and minerals."

Eating well does not guarantee that you are absorbing the
nutrients you need, and that's expecially true for older people,
says Robert M. Russell, M.D., associate professor of medicine
at Tufts and acting director of the Human Nutrition Research
Center on Aging.

Nutrients may be less readily absorbed because stomach-
acid secretion slows down in many older people. In 20 percent
it becomes a potential problem, according to Dr. Russell. It
changes the acid content of the small bowel, where most
nutrients are absorbed, and it prevents foods from breaking
down into particles small enough to be absorbed through the
lining of the bowel. It can inhibit absorption of iron, calcium
and folate, and affect the bacteria in the bowel that produce
vitamin B_{12}.

Unfortunately, the condition is usually symptomless. "Like
high blood pressure, it's silent, with no particular discomfort,"

Dr. Russell says. Severe cases are discovered when the person develops pernicious anemia, a vitamin B_{12}-deficiency disease. Less serious cases are picked up by accident.

There is a simple blood test to detect this condition. It's currently being used only for research but may be commercially available in a few years.

"We know it is a prevalent condition," Dr. Russell says. "What we are trying to pin down right now is just how important this condition is to diagnose because of possible long-term nutritional effects."

And the "cure" may be simple enough. Not necessarily hydrochloric acid drops, which are very sour and unpleasant, but more of whatever nutrients are being affected by this condition.

The Big Picture

"People are always looking for it, but there simply is no single magic bullet or fountain of youth to let us stay young forever," Dr. Blumberg says. Healthy lifestyle and nutrition habits are currently about as close to the magic bullet as we can get. Some of those habits are "negatives"—don't smoke, don't overeat or eat too much fat, don't drink and drive. Others are dos—the positive, active things we can do to stay active and healthy as long as possible. Among those, researchers would list regular exercise, staying mentally active and, of course, good nutrition. "No area has greater potential for improving people's health and well-being," Dr. Blumberg says.

The Vegetarian Edge

Time was when vegetarians were viewed by some as second-class diners, sitting at the lunch counter of life nibbling carrots, tofu and nutburgers while all around them carnivores indulged in a riot of meat and gravy.

Times change, as do attitudes, and today some of those people who once sneered at a meatless diet are wondering if perhaps there's something to vegetarianism after all. Among those wondering are many physicians.

Just glancing at some of the statistics for Seventh-day Adventists, most of whom are vegetarians, is enough to raise the interest of any health-minded person.

A 21-year project that followed the health of more than 25,600 Seventh-day Adventist men and women found that their risk of dying from diabetes is half that of the general population. Looking even closer, researchers found that, especially for men, diabetes was listed more often on the death certificates of meat-eating Adventists than on those of vegetarians. The study's authors offer several theories: Meat or saturated fat may interfere with insulin metabolism; or the relatively low amounts of fiber and complex carbohydrates consumed by meat eaters may enhance their risk of diabetes (*American Journal of Public Health,* May, 1985).

A separate study shows the blood pressure of Seventh-day Adventists to be lower than that of omnivores. Australian scientists found that Adventist men's and women's systolic blood pressure was almost five points lower than nonvegetarians', and the average diastolic blood pressure four to five points lower. The vegetarians were also less likely to be overweight and had lower levels of serum cholesterol, all of which can be risk factors for heart disease (*Australian and New Zealand Journal of Medicine,* August, 1984).

A study of Adventist women also suggests that their vegetarian diet could play a role in preventing the bone-degenerating condition known as osteoporosis that afflicts many postmenopausal women. Medical researchers found that women 50 to 89 years of age who were on a vegetarian diet that included milk and eggs had lost 18 percent bone mineral mass, while women who ate meat had lost 35 percent (*Journal of the American Dietetic Association,* February, 1980).

Since there was little difference in the amount of bone-strengthening calcium the two groups of women consumed over the years, the scientists speculate that meat for some unexplained reason may cause loss of minerals in older women.

English scientists tracked almost 11,000 carnivores and vegetarians for seven years, and found that vegetarians succumbed to heart disease less often, with men faring slightly better than women. The researchers could not conclusively point to a single protective factor in the vegetarians' diet, but suggest that it could be a combination of abstaining from meat, high consumption of other foods, and a health-conscious lifestyle that excludes smoking (*American Journal of Clinical Nutrition,* November, 1982). Researchers at the University of Oxford report that vegetarian women are less likely to develop gallstones. They examined more than 700 women aged 40 to 69 over the course of several years, and noted that the meat-eating women were almost twice as likely to experience problems (*British Medical Journal,* July 6, 1985).

Meanwhile, back in the lab, scientists have been reporting even more benefits of a vegetarian way of eating.

In Sweden, doctors collected patients who were on medication to control high blood pressure and either halted or drastically reduced their usual drug treatments. Instead, the patients exercised and ate a strict vegetarian diet. After one year most of the patients showed a slight decrease in blood pressure, which the researchers hailed as a success, since the reduction was achieved through lifestyle changes. "It would seem, therefore, that the regimen was able to replace this medication," they concluded (*British Journal of Nutrition,* July, 1984).

Hormone Affected

The body of a meat-eating woman processes the female hormone estrogen differently from a vegetarian metabolism. A team of researchers from Boston's New England Medical Center and Tufts University School of Medicine found that vegetarian women excrete two to three times as much estrogen as meat eaters. The more estrogen lost, the lower the levels in the blood. Scientists believe that the recycled estrogen traveling through the bloodstream may have a cancer-linked effect on the breast (*New England Journal of Medicine,* December 16, 1982).

Researchers from Boston's Harvard University Medical School fed vegetarians half a pound of beef a day and watched their pulse rates increase as their cholesterol levels rose 19 percent. The meat portion each vegetarian ate was close to that of the average American's, only leaner. Yet their predicted risk of heart problems increased substantially (*Journal of the American Medical Association,* August 7, 1981).

The vegetarians regained their low cholesterol levels ten days to two weeks after resuming their meatless ways.

It apparently doesn't take long to realize the effects of vegetarianism. A group of omnivores who became experimental vegetarians for a few months realized a decrease in systolic blood pressure of almost seven points and a three-point drop in diastolic pressure. When they resumed eating meat, their blood pressure returned to pretest levels after several weeks (*Lancet,* January, 1983).

Researchers at Loma Linda (California) University School of Medicine have found that vegetarian Seventh-day Adventist men have lower levels of the male hormones testosterone and estradiol. The scientists also note that vegetarian Adventist men eat twice the amount of fiber and have low risks of hormonal-type cancer.

Their theory is that the high-fiber diet may help rid the body of these hormones, which have been linked to prostate cancer (*American Journal of Clinical Nutrition,* July, 1985).

In light of all this, a meat eater who can't bear to part with roast beef may wonder what to do.

"You don't have to adopt a total vegetarian philosophy or lifestyle," says Frank Sacks, M.D., a nutrition researcher at Harvard University Medical School, Boston, who's conducted long-term studies on vegetarian eating. "Reducing your intake of meat and fatty dairy products to only a few times a week will help. If the whole country did this, there'd be a marked decline in heart disease."

Granted, there are other factors that come into play when considering the health status of vegetarians. They generally are concerned about their health and don't smoke or drink to excess, which also has a positive effect. Many of the scientists who've conducted research on meatless eating are quick to acknowledge that lifestyle can play a powerful role.

The ultimate decision rests with the eater. Some will gladly sacrifice a few servings of meat a week in the name of better health.

Others, regardless of what their doctor says is best for

them, will forever consider a plate empty without a piece of meat and declare that green just isn't their color. It's that type of person who usually pulls out the promeat contention that a meal of plants doesn't supply enough protein and is unhealthy. Now, doctors can fall back on the scientific data and politely respond, "Bull."

IF YOU'RE THINKING ABOUT GOING MEATLESS . . .

Whether you're comtemplating a total vegetarian diet or just considering meatless meals a few times a week, a bit of menu planning is in order. Sources of certain nutrients usually obtained from animal foods are listed below.

Nutrient	Sources
Protein	Legumes, grains, nuts and seeds, eggs and dairy products
Calcium	Dairy products, dark leafy greens, legumes, most nuts and seeds, molasses, figs, apricots and dates
Iron	Legumes (especially soybeans and soy products other than oil), dark leafy greens, dried fruits, whole and enriched grains, and molasses
Vitamin B_{12}	Dairy products, eggs, nutritional yeast, foods fortified with B_{12} and supplements
Zinc	Eggs, cheese, legumes, nuts, wheat germ, whole grains and some kinds of brewer's yeast
Riboflavin	Dairy products, eggs, whole and enriched grains, brewer's yeast, dark leafy greens and legumes
Vitamin D	Fortified milk, fortified soy milk, exposure of skin to sunshine

IF YOU'RE THINKING
ABOUT GOING MEATLESS ...
— *Continued*

There are some groups that should take extra care when considering a vegetarian-type diet, according to the American Dietetic Association:

• *Pregnant and lactating women.* Lacto-ovo-vegetarian diets provide all the required nutrients. Iron, folate and zinc supplements may be needed by strict vegetarians.
• *Infants and children.* Lacto-ovo- and ovo-vegetarian (eggs allowed) diets meet the protein requirements for growth, but iron and zinc levels should be watched. Infants on a strict vegan diet should be given fortified soy milk for energy. Deficiencies of calcium, vitamin D, B_{12} and riboflavin easily occur.
• *Adults with special health problems.* Anyone with a diet-related problem, such as lactose intolerance, should consult a professional dietitian for meal planning.

The Super Health Power of Omega-3

Heart disease, rheumatoid arthritis, psoriasis, migraine headaches, breast cancer.

There's a common thread running through this rogues' gallery of modern ills: an unsaturated fat called omega-3. With this thread, scientists hope to unravel the mysteries of some of our most perplexing diseases.

Scientists first became intrigued by omega-3 when they studied the diet of Greenland Eskimos. The Eskimos ate a great deal of fish, much of it very fatty. In fact, Eskimos ate more fat than anyone in the world, yet they suffered virtually no heart disease. The Eskimos' immunity to heart disease was hard to explain. Researchers reasoned that some other factor in the diet might be the key.

They were right. Fish, it turned out, was rich in omega-3, and omega-3 is not just another fish story. Every new study demonstrates the heart-healing properties of this important group of fatty acids. Most medical experts now greet each new bit of information about omega-3 with enthusiasm.

"These highly unsaturated fats seem to give benefit in every study we've reviewed," says William Castelli, M.D., director of the Framingham Heart Study.

Another prominent omega-3 researcher, William E. M. Lands, Ph.D., professor of biological chemistry at the University of Illinois at Chicago, also favors including more fish in the diet.

"The best way to obtain the beneficial omega-3 fatty acids is to eat more seafood," he says. "All the reasons for eating polyunsaturated oils from vegetables remain, certainly. But we need to balance them with omega-3 oils from fish. Omega-3 moderates the body's overutilization of chemicals called eicosanoids formed from polyunsaturates."

One of the prime beneficiaries of a diet high in omega-3 is your heart. That's where the most intensive research has been done. Studies show that omega-3 reduces harmful cholesterol and triglycerides and helps keep arteries clear of blood clots that can cause heart attack or stroke. but scientists recently have been finding other uses for this highly unsaturated fat.

Fishing for Arthritis Relief

One of the most intriguing areas of research involves rheumatoid arthritis.

There is no cure for this painful disease. But some researchers have found that omega-3 fatty acids might offer some relief from the pain and swelling. "We may be recommending omega-3 as an adjunct to traditional therapy in the future," says arthritis researcher Joel M. Kremer, M.D., of Albany Medical College.

A group of eicosanoids called leukotrienes, formed in the body, are thought to cause the characteristic pain and inflammation of rheumatoid arthritis. But omega-3 appears to change the chemical composition of the leukotrienes, making them less inflammatory.

In a study conducted by Dr. Kremer and associates, 23 arthritis patients each were given 1.8 grams of a concentrated fish-oil supplement every day for 12 weeks. Twenty-one other patients received placebos—capsules filled with nothing but wax. As the study progressed, the pain and swelling were reduced in the patients taking supplements. The patients taking placebos showed no improvement (*Lancet,* January 26, 1985). "The results are very encouraging," says Dr. Kremer.

Patients with psoriasis may also benefit from omega-3, since leukotrienes are believed to trigger the characteristic inflammation and scaling of this skin disorder. In British and U.S. studies, omega-3 fatty acids appeared to render leukotrienes less active, resulting in some improvement—but not in all cases. In any event, omega-3 may give some relief from the itching and scaling of psoriasis (*Annals of Allergy,* November, 1985).

Omega-3 also appears to reduce the body's rejection of tissue grafts, though it isn't clear how or why. It's believed graft failure has something to do with the function of blood platelets, which are involved in blood clotting. Tests on laboratory animals show that a diet high in omega-3 reduces tissue-graft failure, presumably by changing the function of the blood platelets (*Journal of Surgical Research,* January, 1986).

Help for Migraines

"The Eskimos have no word in their vocabulary for headache," says Robert J. Hitzemann, Ph.D., associate professor of psychiatry and behavioral sciences at the State University of New York at Stony Brook. All that fish in the Eskimo diet, it seems, can go to your head, too.

One reason why migraine sufferers are predisposed to these unusually painful headaches might be a shortage of eicosapentanoic acid, or EPA, one of the omega-3 fatty acids found in fish. Without EPA, Dr. Hitzemann says, the body releases too much serotonin, a brain chemical that has the capability of either tightening or loosening blood-vessel walls in the brain. All that excess serotonin appears to put the squeeze on blood vessels, resulting in pain.

To test the theory, Dr Hitzemann and his colleagues gave omega-3 supplements to 15 migraine patients. For about half the test subjects, the supplements alleviated pain and resulted in fewer headaches. But all the news wasn't as good, says Dr. Hitzemann. Three of the migraineurs didn't notice any change and four actually became worse.

It's too soon to tell whether eating fish or taking fish-oil supplements can help relieve most migraines, says Dr. Hitzemann, But, he adds, if you've already sought conventional medical advice, it might be worth a try.

"I can't make sweeping recommendations of the basis of a 15-patient study," says Dr. Hitzemann. "Nevertheless, I think we're all convinced this is a breakthrough."

Tumor Prevention

Scientists studying omega-3 also appear to have taken a hopeful step in the battle against breast cancer. Studies linking omega-3 to prevention of breast tumors are still in a very early stage, but they seem to hold promise.

A group of eicosanoids known as prostaglandins lower immunity and encourage tumor growth, says Rashida A. Karmali, Ph.D., associate professor of nutrition at Cook College, Rutgers University.

As a result of an overabundance of these chemicals, says Dr. Karmali, "tumors form faster and the body can't fight them off."

Omega-3 appears to fight off the harmful effects of these overactive chemicals. Dr. Karmali fed fish oil to laboratory rats with breast tumors. The result was a reduction in the number of tumors. "Even when we transplanted tumors from one rat into another, the growth of those established tumors was much slower when we fed them fish oils," she says.

It is one thing to prevent cancer in rats. It is quite another to prevent cancer in people, Dr. Karmali cautions. But the preliminary results of her studies offer some encouragement.

Other studies in the United States tend to support Dr. Karmali's theory.

In one study, conducted at the University of Rochester

School of Medicine, rats fed fish oil developed fewer tumors (*Journal of the National Cancer Institute,* May, 1985).

Researchers at Cornell University had encouraging results, too, when they fed fish oil to laboratory rats. There were fewer tumors and the tumors that did develop were smaller (*Federation Proceedings,* March 1, 1985).

No one can guarantee that eating fish will definitely help prevent breast cancer. But if you want to hedge your bets, Dr. Karmali advises eating more fish or replacing dietary fat with fish-oil supplements.

Back to the Heart

Those potentially harmful eicosanoids, prostaglandins, also know the way to your heart. Simply put, they have a role in making your blood platelets stick to one another, forming floating blood clots.

Where a prostaglandin derivative called thromboxane is telling your platelets to stick together, an omega-3 derivative tells them to break it up and move along. This makes your blood more fluid and reduces the risk that one of those clots—called a thrombus—might find its way into a blood vessel narrowed by atherosclerosis, or hardening of the arteries. The blockage could trigger a heart attack or stroke.

In addition to preventing blood clots from forming, omega-3 fats also seem to help prevent atherosclerosis as well—by influencing cholesterol.

Omega-3 may be very beneficial to people whose cholesterol levels are on the high side—between 230 and 260 milligrams per deciliter of blood. According to Framingham's Dr. Castelli, people with cholesterol levels this high are particularly at risk for heart attack. Despite this, he says, many doctors don't express concern until the levels reach 300 or higher.

"Doctors are missing three-quarters of all the heart attacks in their town by overlooking all the lower numbers," Dr. Castelli says. "The bulk of all our heart attacks occur at cholesterol levels between 230 and 260. If you do not lower cholesterol, you will not have a favorable effect on heart disease."

One way to lower your cholesterol, says Dr. Castelli, is simply to eat more fish.

In one recent study at Vanderbilt University School of Medicine, in Nashville, patients took about three tablespoons of an omega-3-rich fish-oil supplement every day. At the end of the four-week study, serum cholesterol was reduced by 15 percent (*Internal Medicine News,* January 15-31, 1986).

Adding Fish to Your Diet

You don't have to eat as much fish as the Eskimos do to decrease your risks of heart disease, cancer and other illnesses. Experts think we might prevent disease by eating comparatively little.

Most researchers believe as few as two to four fish meals a week might be sufficient. The more you eat, obviously, the better.

"The ideal amount to eat probably varies from person to person," says William E. Connor, M.D., professor of medicine at the Oregon Health Sciences University and one of the pioneers in omega-3 research. "A couple of six-ounce fish meals a week is probably the minimum. I certainly enjoy three to four servings of fish a week."

Of course, Dr. Connor adds, you ought to watch your weight, keep your blood pressure under control, avoid stress, eat fewer saturated fats and stop smoking. "The omega-3 theory is a tremendous advance," Dr. Conner told a symposium audience in March. "But there are other basic things to consider."

Most experts agree that fish should be substituted for red meat and poultry and not eaten in addition to what you normally consume. The meat we get from farm animals is low in omega-3.

Not all fish contain the same amount of omega-3 (see table). Generally, fattier fish—sardines, salmon and mackerel, for example—contain more. Ocean fish have more than fresh-water fish. Shellfish, too, contain considerable omega-3.

If you don't like fish, supplements may be a alternative.

HOW MUCH OMEGA-3 IS THERE IN YOUR FISH?

Here are some of the best sources of omega-3 in fish.

Fish	Grams per 3½-Oz. Serving
Sardines, Norway	5.1
Salmon, chinook	3.04
Mackerel, Atlantic	2.18
Salmon, pink	1.87
Tuna, albacore*	1.69
Sablefish	1.39
Herring, Atlantic	1.09
Trout, rainbow (U.S.)	1.08
Oysters, Pacific	.84
Striped bass	.64
Catfish, channel	.61
Alaska king crab	.57
Perch, ocean	.51
Blue crab†	.46
Halibut, Pacific	.45
Shrimp, different species	.39
Flounder, yellowtail	.30
Haddock	.16

*Canned, light
†Cooked, canned

SOURCES: Adapted from
Journal of the American Dietetic Association, vol. 69 and 71.
"Omega-3: Food for a Healthy Heart," Norway Sardine Industry.

Ten capsules of concentrated marine lipids supply 1.8 grams of eicosapentanoic acid, or EPA, one of the omega-3 components. A serving of salmon (about four ounces) contains about a gram of EPA. Cod-liver oil, too, contains EPA, but the amount varies according to brand. Cod-liver oil usually contains high amounts of vitamins A and D, however, and in large amounts these can be toxic, so cod-liver oil should not be used for this purpose.

Is Your Body Too Dry?

Chances are you don't think too much about water until it's not there when you want it. Then, it doesn't take long to regret having taken it for granted. After about three days without water, you'd be plenty sorry. In a week, more or less, you'd be too dried up to care.

You don't have to be staked to an anthill in the Sahara to experience dehydration, however. It is an insidious process, and more common than most realize. You can be pregnant, sweating heavily or taking certain medications. Or, you may be older and have undetected diabetes, a weak thirst response or slowed kidney function.

And your symptoms may be varied. You could be weak, light-headed, flushed, intolerant of heat, irritable or confused. If you're an athlete, you might notice your performance is lagging, or that you're getting muscle cramps.

It's true that most of us need not be concerned about dehydration. If we sweat or urinate too much, our bodies quickly respond. Cells in the brain sense a drop in blood volume and an increase in the salt levels of the blood. They excrete a biochemical that makes us thirsty. At the same time, other cells put out a biochemical that makes the kidneys conserve water. We urinate a darker, more concentrated fluid.

In healthy younger people these two mechanisms work just fine to keep the right amount of water in our bodies. We drink exactly enough to restore the normal concentration of molecules of salt in our blood. Or, if we overdrink, our kidneys soon dump the excess.

But it's also true that some people need to watch how much water they drink, because their body's monitoring system is faulty. They may not be drinking enough. Or, in rare cases, they may be getting too much.

Thirst Mechanism Slows

Researchers have found that healthy older people whose bodies need water are not likely to feel thirsty the way younger people do. Deprived of water for 24 hours, older people are less likely to say they feel thirsty or to complain of a dry mouth, even though their blood samples show they are actually more dehydrated. The older folks also fill up on less when they drink again (*New England Journal of Medicine,* September 20, 1984).

"These findings suggest that older people can't rely on their thirst mechanism to determine how much water they should be drinking," says the study's main researcher, Barbara Rolls, Ph.D., of Johns Hopkins University School of Medicine, Baltimore. Combine this with the aging kidney's inability to conserve water and you've got the potential for a real problem.

"If they are sick, in the hospital, on medication, or get diarrhea, older people face the danger of becoming seriously dehydrated because they do not ask for fluids," Dr. Rolls says.

Dehydration is serious business. Our bodies are 60 percent water, which means there's water, water, everywhere, from the thick jelly inside our eyeballs to the fluid in which our brains float. The initial effect of dehydration is a decrease in blood volume. The blood thickens as the ratio of plasma to blood cells decreases, the heart must pump more vigorously, and we end up with what's known as circulatory insufficiency. We also tend to overheat, as the body's main cooling systems work to conserve fluid. Eventually, as the body continues to draw water out of the cells trying to restore blood volume and cool itself, we could literally dry up and die.

Mild dehydration can cause weariness, loss of appetite, flushed skin, heat intolerance, impatience, indistinct speech, stumbling and dizziness. More severe symptoms include muscle spasms, delirium, shriveled skin, inability to swallow, sunken eyes, dim vision, painful urination, deafness and numb skin. Severe dehydration ends in seizures, coma and death.

Diabetes can cause dehydration in older people. In this disease, the kidneys use up lots of water to filter sugar out of the blood. In younger people, this larger urine output produces increased thirst, a symptom that alerts doctors to check for early diabetes.

"But older people who have developed diabetes do not always report symptoms of thirst to their doctors, which may be one reason they are not diagnosed," Dr. Rolls says.

Diuretics Can Dry You Out

Diuretics are potent drugs that draw salt and water from your body. They are often used to control high blood pressure or to relieve edema—water-logged tissues caused by hormone imbalances or heart or kidney failure. These drugs are meant to dry you out. The problem is that the careful monitoring of dosage that is needed to avoid problems often is not provided.

"Commonly, patients are started on a high dose to relieve edema," says William Kaehny, M.D., a kidney-disease specialist and associate professor of medicine at the University of Colorado School of Medicine, Denver. "Once the edema is gone, the dose should be decreased." That's not always done, and the result is dehydration.

"Blood volume and, so, blood pressure decrease, so when you stand up you get light-headed and may even faint," Dr. Kaehny says. "You may have muscle cramps, nausea, even vomiting if your blood pressure gets low enough."

If you're taking diuretics, it's important to have your blood pressure checked both lying down and standing, Dr. Kaehny says. "Your blood volume may be fine lying down, but when you stand and blood pools in your legs, it may not be enough." Check with your doctor about cutting back on your diuretic dosage.

During a heat wave, diuretics can greatly increase your risks of dehydration, warn two British researchers. They found this out when they decided to increase the diuretic dosage of an 86-year-old woman whose ankles had become badly swollen during unusually hot weather. After three weeks on the medicine, the woman became mentally confused and kept falling down.

Her condition, although serious, was easily remedied by replenishing her body with salt and water. Diuretics are frequently used drugs in the elderly, the doctors note. They recommend diuretic dosages be reduced or stopped altogether during heat waves (*Lancet,* October 22, 1983).

How Much Should You Drink?

Simply telling people to drink more water may be good enough advice for most, but it isn't specific enough for very old or ill people, Dr. Rolls says. Most people do well with 1½ to 2 quarts of fluid a day—six to eight eight-ounce glasses of liquid or less, depending on the amount of fluid they get from foods. But some need to drink more, and some get by well on less.

"People's kidneys vary greatly in how much water they conserve," Dr. Rolls says. She suggests you periodically check the color of your urine to make sure it's moderately dilute. If it seems concentrated—if the color is dark or the odor is strong—increase the amount of liquids you drink.

If you live in or visit a dry, hot climate, your water needs increase dramatically. You sweat more, but since the sweat quickly evaporates, you may not notice how much water you are losing. Dry wind, hot or cold, also dries you out as effectively as it dries sheets on a clothesline.

Athletes would do well to drink half a cup or more of water before they start their game or race, and to frequently drink small amounts during their activity, sports-medicine specialists agree. Muscle cramps that occur after a period of exertion are frequently due to dehydration.

Plain Water Still Seems Best

The debate continues on what kind of fluids are best to drink, with plain water still getting the most votes. Avoid very sugary drinks if you're dry, the American College of Sports Medicine recommends. Sugar drinks are absorbed into the body much more slowly than plain water. And even though that cold beer goes down easy, don't make it your first choice for thirst quenching. Alcohol has a diuretic effect, releasing fluids from your body just when it is craving fluids the most.

It's true that your body does lose salt in sweat, but the amounts are very small. You may want to replenish yourself, though, with a lightly salted broth or vegetable soup if you're recovering from a serious bout of diarrhea or vomiting, Dr. Kaehny suggests. Such intestinal eruptions deplete sodium and other minerals, such as potassium, magnesium and calcium, which may all play roles in water balance.

There are cases where you'll be told to drink beyond the call of thirst.

People prone to kidney stones are often advised to drink more water. "And it works," Dr. Kaehny says. "Drinking about four quarts of fluid a day markedly reduces the formation of all kinds of kidney stones." Water dilutes the minerals that can crystalize in the kidney, forming stones.

Some drugs can also form crystals in the kidney, damaging the tiny tubules that filter the blood. Sulfa drugs (antibacterial agents prescribed for problems like bladder infections) and some chemotherapy drugs are the most likely offenders. "If the label on a drug says to drink plenty of fluids, make sure you do that," Dr. Kaehny warns. Drinking plenty of water with a medicine also allows you to absorb more of it, and reduces the possibility of irritation to your throat or stomach.

Bladder infections also benefit from forced drinking. "The water flushes bacteria and inflammatory debris from the bladder," Dr. Kaehny says. You might not want to worry about getting up at night for a drink, though. Researchers have found that highly concentrated urine, like that found in the bladder after a long night's sleep, helps slow bacterial growth.

Too Much of a Good Thing?

Most of us would have to work darn hard to guzzle so much water that we develop "water intoxication"—with symptoms of drunkenness that can lead to death as brain cells expand with fluid, then burst. But there are some instances of too much of a good thing, however rare these cases might be.

A California doctor, for instance, notes that he has recently seen three women who had epileptic fits as a result of a high-water diet. Their epilepsy had been controlled with medication, but after following a diet plan that advocated drinking 8 to 12 eight-ounce glasses of water a day, they suddenly began to have seizures (*New England Journal of Medicine,* January 24, 1985).

And a woman who drank 30 glasses of water, one right after another, in a misguided effort to prepare herself for an ultrasound test, lapsed into unconsciousness hours later. Luckily, her mother told doctors about all the water she had drunk.

An intravenous salt solution flushed the excess fluid from the woman's body and she was well (and, hopefully, wiser) four days later (*European Neurology,* number 4, 1985).

Something as cheap and available as water may be overlooked as a cure, or cause, of an illness. But it could be the simplest medicine ever devised, short of breathing. So treat your body as well as you do your houseplants—water it regularly.

The Healing Power of Fruit

Fruit is one of the most healthful foods that can cross your lips. It's rich in vitamins, minerals and fiber that have been shown to help protect against everything from cancer to dental dilemmas to the common cold. Fruit's low in calories, salt and fat.

One of the most significant pieces of recent evidence favoring fresh fruit comes from the Orient, where researchers from the American Cancer Society enrolled more than 1 million Japanese in a study that spanned 11 years. The objective was to see if fruit, fruit juice, green salad or vitamin supplements had any effect on lung cancer caused by cigarette smoking.

The results, which focus on males only since the majority of Japanese smokers are men, show that those who ate fresh fruit five to seven days a week were less likely to get lung cancer. The smokers who dined on fruit three or four days a week, however, were 25 percent more likely to die from cancer. Those who avoided fruit completely or ate it only one or two days a week were 75 percent more likely to succumb to the disease (*Chinese Medical Journal,* March, 1985).

Fruit juice had similar protective effects, but green salad had "little or no influence upon lung cancer," they report, adding that "frequently taking multivitamin pills cannot substitute for eating fruit or drinking fruit juice, although they often contain vitamins A and C."

The Japanese study is just one chapter in the book of fruit's benefits. Ancel Keys, Ph.D., a well-known medical researcher and professor emeritus from the University of Minnesota, has also contributed. He was among the first to recognize the health advantages of the so-called Mediterranean diet, which is now being espoused as a way to stay healthy. In studies of the working-class people of Naples, Italy, he found low blood-cholesterol levels, few problems with excess weight, and only rare cases of coronary heart disease. Besides other dietary habits that have a positive influence, such as eating a lot of vegetables and complex carbohydrates, Dr. Keys found that their diets always included fresh fruit for dessert and none of the rich, sugary, after-meal treats so popular in his homeland.

What follows are several of the more pressing health concerns of our time and the influence fruit may have on each.

High Blood Pressure

Fresh fruit has little, if any, sodium, which means it's ideal for people concerned about their blood pressure. A glass of milk, which isn't considered a high-salt food, contains 126 milligrams of sodium, while half a cantaloupe offers 23 milligrams, a large peach has less than 1 milligram and a two-pound watermelon only 4 milligrams.

One thing fruit does have is potassium. Researchers have found that people whose diets are high in potassium—vegetarians, for instance—have a low incidence of high blood pressure, even if they're genetically predisposed to the condition and don't control their salt intake. So instead of just avoiding many foods because of a possible negative agent, hypertensives can help themselves to fruit and this positive nutrient.

Many fresh fruits are excellent sources of potassium: A banana offers 451 milligrams, one-quarter of a cantaloupe 413 milligrams and three apricots 313 milligrams. A good summer cooler is half a cantaloupe filled with low-fat ice milk, or a drink made of orange juice (one cup has 496 milligrams of potassium), bananas and nonfat dry milk mixed in a blender.

Heart Disease

It's widely known that the best road to heart disease is a high-fat diet. And fresh fruit is perfect for a low-fat snack or meal. You'd have to eat 9½ pounds of cherries to get the same amount of fat found in one ounce of potato chips.

In addition, fruit contains pectin, a type of fiber that may help prevent heart disease. While it's uncertain exactly how pectin works, some researchers say the fiber captures excess cholesterol in the digestive tract and flushes it out of the body before it can be reabsorbed. Others say the fiber selectively raises the level of HDL cholesterol, the good kind that is correlated with a decrease in heart disease.

The vitamin C found in fresh fruit may help reduce levels of cholesterol in the blood, a risk factor for atherosclerosis and heart attack. For the past 30 years, some scientists have been reporting that vitamin C lowers cholesterol levels in humans and protects laboratory animals from atherosclerosis. It's believed vitamin C can help promote the transformation of cholesterol to bile acids, which can then be excreted from the body.

Unfortunately, man, guinea pigs and other primates can't synthesize the nutrient within the body and must depend on external sources, which is why fruit is so important. One orange supplies more than the Recommended Dietary Allowance (RDA) of vitamin C for an adult, and most other fruits—limes, lemons, apricots, strawberries and cantaloupes, among others—will handily contribute to the RDA.

Cancer

Regular helpings of fresh fruit also supply you with beta-carotene, a naturally occurring pigment that gives many fruits and vegetables their green or yellow hue. It's also been linked to cancer prevention. Found in apricots, mangoes, peaches, watermelons, even cherries and apples, beta-carotene is converted by the body into vitamin A. The big question is whether beta-carotene or vitamin A protects against cancer.

"We're not sure, but we suspect it's the beta-carotene," says Fred Khachik, Ph.D., who researches carotenoids in fruits and vegetables for the U.S. Department of Agriculture's Agricultural Research Service, Human Nutrition Research Center in Beltsville, Maryland. "There are other carotenoids in fruit which are not converted into vitamin A. They could also be responsible or working in combination with beta-carotene and possibly some micronutrients. We can say, however, that there's definitely a relationship between foods with beta-carotene and cancer prevention."

It's suspected that beta-carotene protects cells from free

radicals, by-products of fat metabolism that can turn a healthy cell cancerous. Whatever the reason, the evidence favoring fruits with beta-carotene is mounting:

● In Japan, people whose daily diets included foods containing beta-carotene were less likely to develop lung, stomach and other cancers. The ongoing study, which so far has spanned 20 years, also shows that the damage caused by bad habits, such as smoking or avoiding fruits for years, is reversible (*Dietary Aspects of Carcinogenesis,* September, 1983).

● A team of scientists from the National Cancer Institute in Bethesda, Maryland, found that women who eat foods containing beta-carotene are less likely to develop mouth or throat cancer. A study of 227 women who had these types of cancer revealed that those who ate 21 or more servings of fresh fruit—and vegetables—a week cut their risk in half. The researchers reported that those who ate moderate amounts—11 to 20 servings a week—reduced their chances by about 35 percent (*Cancer Research,* volume 44, March, 1984).

The vitamin C in fresh fruit may also protect against nitrosamines, cancer-causing agents that form when common food additives called nitrites interact with body chemicals. The nutrient apparently combines with nitrites in the stomach to hinder their transformation into carcinogens. Since nitrites are present in foods only in small amounts, it's believed that an orange eaten with the meal will suffice. Ideally, the vitamin C should be consumed just before dining so it's waiting in the stomach for the potential carcinogens.

Blood Sugar

Fresh fruit contains natural sugars (predominantly fructose) that provide energy without too rapid a rise in blood-sugar levels, which can occur after eating foods with more concentrated sugars. A drastic change in blood-sugar levels can cause problems for diabetics or hypoglycemics.

"When fruit fiber reaches the stomach, passage of the meal into the intestines is slowed. A gel-like substance, formed from certain fibers such as pectin, coats the intestinal lining," says Sheldon Reiser, Ph.D., head of carbohydrate research at the USDA's human nutrition branch. This protective coating slows the absorption of glucose, a natural product of the digestive process. Keeping glucose in check is important because wild swings in glucose levels cause insulin levels to react similarly, which can lead to problems.

Researchers in England report similar fruit-fiber findings. When volunteers were fed whole oranges and also juice, their insulin levels jumped dramatically after drinking the juice, but slowly after ingesting the fruit pieces. Citing previous studies with whole apples and juice that produced similar results, the scientists conclude that while the glucose content of the fruit obviously influences blood-sugar levels, fiber apparently helps keep glucose and insulin levels from bouncing around unhealthily (*American Journal of Clinical Nutrition,* February, 1981).

Fruit fiber also leaves you feeling full longer than most foods and may help with weight loss. The gel that coats the intestinal tract and slows glucose absorption also helps slow the meal as it moves through the digestive tract. Because fruit fiber lingers inside longer than most foods, it may leave you feeling fuller longer, and forestall those hunger pangs that are the downfall of so many dieters.

"It seems logical that you won't get hungry as soon as you would after eating foods that empty out of your system faster, such as cookies and brownies," says Dr. Reiser.

The English researchers who undertook the orange study found the same. Both oranges and apples left people feeling fuller and "the return of appetite was delayed," they report.

While unsure of whether it was the fruits' bulk or fiber that caused the fullness, they note that turning apples into a drinkable puree reduced the feeling somewhat.

Most important for the weight conscious, fruit is low in calories, and ounce for ounce you can eat more and get fewer calories.

There are 235 calories in a piece of chocolate cake, compared to 94 calories in half a cantaloupe filled with strawberries and topped with yogurt.

For those who need even more prodding toward the fresh fruit market, consider some of the other pluses that await:

● *folacin,* an essential B vitamin needed for the maturation of red blood cells

● *vitamin B₆,* crucial for protein metabolism (one medium-size banana supplies half of the adult RDA)
● *magnesium,* a catalyst in several hundred biological reactions (a cup of fresh blackberries provides about 10 percent of the RDA).

Besides the already-mentioned benefits of vitamin C, that nutrient has been shown to help: cure gum disease and also improve the eyesight of people suffering from glaucoma; accelerate healing after injury or surgery, and reduce recovery time by 50 to 75 percent; and strengthen the immune system so a cold may not last as long.

Yet, even in the face of such strong evidence in fresh fruit's behalf, there's still one perplexing question: why some people, when given a choice between a candy bar and a piece of fruit, invariably reach for the chocolate?

"It's been shown that infants are born with a preference for sweet things, which is often carried over into adulthood, unless habits change along the way," says Wendy Gasch, a nutritionist and registered dietitian with the International Life Sciences Institute-Nutrition Foundation, Washington, D.C. "But in the case of dietary habits, it's never too late to make a change, especially when it's such a good change."

Protecting and Restoring Your Good Health

How to Keep Out of a Germ's Flight Path

We worry about catching a cold from the bathroom rinsing glass and cold sores from the pay phone. And who knows what microbial assassins lie in wait among the stiff, unyielding folds of bubblegum stuck to the bottom of the seat in the movies or in that wadded mass of tissue paper wedged into the nozzle of the drinking fountain?

Though you *can* catch a cold or flu from an inanimate object, doctors suggest we have more to fear from person-to-person contact.

This is not to say illness is transmitted only by people. Disease-causing organisms in the environment do take their toll. The bacterium that causes Legionnaires' disease, for example, was found to live in air-conditioning cooling towers and in various sources of fresh water.

Even though a disease may originate somewhere outside the human environment—one type of influenza virus may reside in swine, for instance—humans are more adept at spreading disease.

To better understand what you can and cannot catch—and how—it helps to take a closer look at viruses. They take on many forms and cause a variety of illnesses, from the common cold to the dreaded disease AIDS.

The Common Cold

How does that cold virus find its way from someone else's red nose to yours?

Cold viruses attack the upper respiratory tract. When cold sufferers sneeze or cough, they spray extremely fine droplets of virus-bearing mucus and saliva into their environment. Whether you are felled by a sneeze depends on how big (or how small) the droplets, the distance between you and the sneezer—and time.

"There's no such thing as a dry sneeze," says Albert Balows, Ph.D., assistant director for laboratory sciences at the Centers for Disease Control in Atlanta. "The smaller the droplets are, the greater the trajectory they have and the longer they float in air."

The longer the droplets remain on the floor, the less potent they become. When they dry, the virus dies.

How long can a cold virus live outside the body?

According to Jack Gwaltney, M.D., head of epidemiology and virology at the University of Virginia School of Medicine, the viruses associated with colds can live outside the body for hours or even days. The rhinovirus in particular can survive up to five days.

If you didn't catch your cold from airborne particles drifting by at the bus stop, it's conceivable you caught it from an environmental object—what researchers call fomites.

Among the fomites, however, the most likely culprit is not a coffee cup, a telephone or a public drinking fountain—it's the hand of a person who has a cold.

"There's some evidence, with rhinovirus in particular, that you are apt to have the virus on your hands," says Dr. Gwaltney. Ironically, people who considerately cough or sneeze into a tissue to avoid spreading their cold often wind up with the virus on their hands as mucus seeps through the paper. Clinical tests have demonstrated that a person with cold viruses on his hand can directly infect another person, Dr. Gwaltney says.

This shouldn't discourage you from continuing to shield the innocent from your explosive sneezes. However, Dr. Gwaltney recommends washing your hands frequently when you have a cold or are in the presence of a cold sufferer.

There's at least one virus for every person living in Zwingle, Iowa (population 119 at last count)—with plenty of bugs to spare. Therein lies the root of our vulnerability.

"Because there are so many different cold-causing viruses—in excess of 100—a person can develop a cold from virus number one and, following recovery, may develop an immunity that will protect that person for some time," says Dr. Balows. "But it doesn't give him a nickel's worth of protection from virus number two."

If you don't have a cold, your best bet for preventing one is staying away from those who do, although that's easier said than done.

In the meantime, the search for a cold cure—a search some researchers consider an impossible dream—goes on. Among the proposed remedies: interferon, a natural antiviral substance produced in the body, now being reproduced in quantity in the laboratory.

Herpes Simplex Virus

From the cold virus, which comes and goes over about a week's time, we proceed to viruses considerably more obstinate.

Herpes simplex comes in two varieties. Herpes 1 usually is associated with distinctive, crusty cold sores on the lips. Type 2 usually causes painful sores in the genital area.

Herpes of both varieties are easily transmissible. In fact, says Dr. Balows, there is evidence herpes—particularly the oral variety—is present in the bodies of most human beings from an early age.

"They're both related and have a number of characteristics in common. Herpes is unusual in that the virus, particularly type 1, is acquired by almost every human in the early stages of life and doesn't produce any lesions."

Even if herpes is hiding out inside your body, you might live your entire life without a sore. The outward symptoms of herpes can be triggered, however, by stress of almost any type and through fever-producing illness.

"Herpes virus has the unusual ability to hole up in the nerve ganglia. They just get into nerve tissue cells and 'hibernate' there. They can hibernate there a lifetime," according to Dr. Balows.

Herpes of both varieties are transmitted by personal contact. While most cases of herpes type 1 occur on the mouth, lips and nostrils and cases of herpes type 2 on the genital organs, we now know that type 2 may cause oral outbreaks and type 1 may cause sores in the genital area in a small number of cases.

Herpes is transmitted by close body contact—kissing, intercourse, oral or anal sex. The virus lives exclusively in humans.

If you are concerned about catching herpes 1 or 2 from someone who has it, it's important to know that the viruses are transmitted only when there are active sores. When the viruses are dormant, says Dr. Balows, it is "virtually impossible" to spread the disease.

Not everyone who is exposed to the viruses will develop symptoms. "For reasons that are not totally understood, some individuals are more susceptible than others," says Dr. Balows.

Can you catch herpes from an environmental source? Is it possible to contract genital herpes from a toilet seat in a public restroom, for example? The odds of such a transmission are extremely low.

Trudy Larson, M.D., and Yvonne Bryson, M.D., of the UCLA School of Medicine, conducted a study in which a herpes type-2 patient sat on a plastic toilet seat. The patient's sores were on the backs of his thighs.

The study showed that the virus survived an hour and a half.

However, according to Dr. Bryson, "It would be very unlikely you would catch it that way." For one thing, she says herpes 2 sores usually are found on and about the genitals and, less frequently, on the buttocks or the thighs. Furthermore, for a second person to contract the virus, the skin of that person's thighs or buttocks probably would have to be broken. "Skin is a good barrier," says Dr. Bryson. "Herpes 2 doesn't penetrate intact skin."

For the genitals to come into contact with the deposit, a person would have to be sitting on the seat in an unusual way.

Dr. Bryson's verdict on toilet-seat transmission of herpes: "It's not a real public health hazard. We have no documented cases of transmission in this fashion."

It's possible to transmit herpes type 1—oral herpes—to the eyes by touching the eyes with your fingers after they've come into contact with the herpes-infected mouth. People who wear contact lenses, for example, are vulnerable, those who wet their lenses with saliva in particular. Herpes in the eye—ocular herpes—can cause blindness. People who wear contact lenses need to be instructed to maintain strict discipline in the removal, cleansing and sterilization of their lenses. "It has to be a procedure that's followed virtually like a religious doctrine," says Dr. Balows.

As for those who persist in wetting their lenses with saliva, he adds, "They're asking for it. They're just red-hot candidates for ocular herpes. It's unusual but it should never exist."

A final note: Herpes can be transmitted to a newborn during childbirth. The result, often, is death.

Viruses from active genital herpes sores in the mother find their way into the baby's bloodstream and, ultimately, into the brain, causing herpes encephalitis. Doctors can't do much to prevent an outbreak of genital herpes in the mother but, to reduce the risk, babies born to these mothers frequently are delivered by cesarean section.

Is there a way to avoid catching herpes? If your mate is suffering through an outbreak of oral herpes, kissing is, or should be, verboten. In simulated testing, intact condoms have been shown to provide an effective physical barrier against herpes 2. However, doctors still recommend abstinence when herpes sores are present.

If you have genital herpes, a relatively new drug, acyclovir, has been demonstrated effective in reducing the pain of herpes and shortening the period of the virus's activity. Long-term progress is being made on a vaccine to prevent herpes in those who have not had the disease, but such a vaccine probably won't help those who already have herpes.

AIDS

The virus that causes Acquired Immune Deficiency Syndrome is far more insidious than the herpes viruses or any one of the viruses that cause colds. The virus in question has a name: human T cell lymphotropic virus, or HTLV-III for short. HTLV-III attacks white blood cells called T4 lymphocytes. These cells, derived from the thymus gland, play a key role in our body's defenses against infection and disease.

HTLV-III has a voracious appetite for T cells. It hijacks the cells, forces them to stop doing what they normally do, and demands that the cells reproduce more viruses like itself.

"When it has utilized its substance within the cell, the lymphocyte shrivels up, the virus escapes and invades other T4 cells," says CDC's Dr. Balows. As a result of this systematic cell wipeout, the host—the virus's human victim—is deprived of immunity. Consequently, the victim is susceptible to any one of a number of infections that would not normally present a challenge to the immune system.

"Organisms already in the body will take advantage of this to overgrow," says Dr. Balows. "It's like a weed in your yard. Over time it will kill the host."

About 80 percent of those who develop AIDS can be expected to die. There is, as yet, no cure for AIDS, which afflicts homosexuals, intravenous drug abusers, blood-transfusion recipients and heterosexuals who increasingly are coming into contact with the virus through contact with bisexuals.

There's another, related malady called AIDS-related complex. This simply means that a person carries the virus, but his body is, essentially, holding its own against the invader. Over time, ARC could progress to a full-blown case of AIDS, remain essentially unchanged, or appear to improve for reasons unknown.

This doesn't mean the virus goes away. In fact, it appears to remain dormant in the body.

By the same token, there's a percentage of people who are

AIDS infected but who don't show signs of the disease. "We don't know yet what this means," says Dr. Balows.

AIDS is contagious. How do you catch it? Primarily through sexual contact between homosexuals and, to a limited degree, through heterosexual contact with infected bisexual partners. Among intravenous drug abusers, the disease spreads as a result of shared needles. Drug abusers have low resistance to disease, in any case.

Those who worry about getting AIDS from a blood transfusion should know that there now is a test administered to blood donors that effectively screens out AIDS-infected individuals. For hemophiliacs, who also were considered at risk, the threat has been substantially minimized by means of a new process in which the clotting factor hemophiliacs need to live is heated, killing the AIDS virus.

Dr. Balows says he expects blood-transfusion-transmitted AIDS to decrease "as long as we keep up our guard."

Those more at risk are highly sexually active homosexuals. "That level of promiscuity just increases the risk of exposure," says Dr. Balows. Homosexuals can reduce the risk by a change in lifestyle—fewer sex partners and greater selectivity, perhaps even monogamy.

According to Dr. Balows, there is no evidence at this time that AIDS can be transmitted through fomites. Many who are likely to come in contact with potential AIDS carriers—doctors, nurses, barbers, ambulance attendants, undertakers and so on—have expressed concern, however.

Should the paramedic worry about mouth-to-mouth resuscitation? Should the barber toss away his brush and comb? Should the undertaker take extraordinary care in embalming the corpse of an AIDS victim?

"All we can tell them is to do as you normally would," recommends Dr. Balows. "You don't have to throw away your comb and brush." As for undertakers, if they follow the usual scientific procedures in embalming the body, there should be no problem.

The AIDS virus has been found to be present in saliva, though there's no evidence that it can be transmitted by kissing, even passionate kissing. But Dr. Balows doesn't recommend it. "It just stands to reason, if you know there's a tiger in the cage, you just don't walk into the cage," he says.

Can you get AIDS from mouth-to-mouth resuscitation? "You can't give out written guarantees that you can't transmit it through mouth-to-mouth, but it's so unlikely as not to create a risk group," says Dr. Balows.

Is a vaccine on the way? Research is progressing, but there have been no definitive results. In any event, a vaccine would be useful in preventing AIDS, but probably wouldn't help those already suffering.

Infectious or Not?

Here is a brief rundown on the "catch-factors" of more common health problems:

Acne ● Acne is not catching. It's genetic, and stress of all kinds may trigger an outbreak in susceptible individuals. Chocolate has little or nothing to do with it, experts insist.

Athlete's Foot ● The fungus among us can cause the itching, burning and scaling known as athlete's foot.

Is it catching? Yes, but not for everybody. Dermatologists say some of us get athlete's foot while others resist the pesky dermatophytes, for reasons not clearly understood. Bacteria also play a role in bringing about the peeling and blisters of athlete's foot.

Athlete's foot fungi like a moist environment. For this reason, the floor of the locker-room shower stall and shoes that encourage profuse sweating—sneakers that don't permit the foot to "breathe," for instance—may be perfect breeding grounds for athlete's foot fungi. Topical ointments have been shown to be effective in banishing the fungi from between your toes, but not in preventing athlete's foot.

Canker Sores ● These painful mouth ulcers are not contagious. They are caused by injuries to the mouth. Some studies indicate that there may be links to stress.

Eczema ● The root cause of this itchy skin disease remains unknown. You can't catch eczema from someone else. Remedies—not cures—range from topical steroids to cold cloths to diet therapy to a change of climate.

Herpes Zoster ● Also known as shingles, herpes zoster consists of fever, along with a painful rash, most of the time between the neck and the abdomen. It isn't contagious. Herpes zoster is not a sexually transmitted disease, but rather an illness triggered by the chicken-pox virus, acquired in childhood. The virus emerges from dormancy to cause the characteristic body rash.

Experts believe the awakening of the once-sleeping virus is related to lapses in our immunity. For this reason, herpes zoster outbreaks become more common as people grow older.

Hot-Tub Trouble ● The warm, moist environment of the spa is a disease bug's playground. The herpes virus can survive up to 4½ hours on a plastic spa seat or bench, for instance. Although rare, it is also possible to catch pneumonia by inhaling superfine water droplets contaminated with *Pseudomonas aeruginosa* bacteria. The same bug can cause "hot-tub dermatitis," swimmer's ear and urinary-tract infections. The bacteria flourish in inadequately chlorinated hot tubs.

Strep Throat ● This bacterial infection, characterized by a sore, red throat and high temperature, is catching. Untreated, it can lead to rheumatic fever.

The infection is transmitted by direct or indirect personal contact. Another, less well publicized mode of transmission is inadequately refrigerated food. The adaptable bacteria also are known to cause skin infections ("scrum strep") in athletes who participate in contact sports.

Toilet Terrors ● Use care when using the toilet. Urine infected with the *trichomonas* protozoa has been proved to splash upward onto the genitalia of women, sometimes causing trichomoniasis.

Trench Mouth ● You can't catch trench mouth, though you may share certain predisposing factors in common with others who get it. The bacteria that cause trench mouth are thought to be present in many people, yet only a small percentage suffer with the periodic mouth ulcers and pain, with outbreaks usually associated with stress or illness. Interestingly, one study suggests trench mouth is much more likely to affect whites than blacks.

Warts ● You can't catch warts from a frog, but you can get warts from another person. Warts are caused by a virus, which enters the skin of the susceptible person through a cut or scratch. To catch warts, your immune system defenses must be lowered, generally through illness. Certain prescription drugs—drugs used to treat allergies, for instance—can have the same effect.

Wart viruses can be picked up by direct contact with an infected person or indirectly in moist environments such as showers or swimming pools.

Rounding Out Your Breast Protection Plan

If there's one thing that cancer research is making clear, it's that far fewer people could be dying from this disease than currently do. As researchers unravel cancer's complexities, they've been discovering sensible, easy ways people can protect themselves from this deadly disease. Some of the latest, and best, of these practical research findings in breast cancer and benign breast disease are presented here.

Perhaps you've avoided having your breasts screened for cancer by mammography because you fear that radiation from this x-ray technique could cause the cancer it's meant to detect. If so, it's time to put those worries aside, permanently.

The amount of radiation used in today's standard mammography (called xeromammography) is about one-tenth what it was 20 years ago. It's less than two rads of exposure.

"The radiation risk today is so small there literally is no risk," says Leon Speroff, M.D., chairman of the department of reproductive biology at Case Western Reserve University, Cleveland. An even newer form of mammography, the film-screen technique, available at larger city hospitals, uses the lowest dose of radiation ever—one-tenth of a rad.

Indeed, you may face more risk by not having mammograms done regularly as you grow older. Recent large-scale, long-term studies are showing mammography to be a highly effective way to prevent deaths from breast cancer through early detection. In the Netherlands, annual mammographic screening reduced risk of breast-cancer death among women age 35 or over by 50 percent in one city.

The first reports from a long-term study in Sweden may show even more positive results. In this ongoing study, 162,981 women were randomly put into one of two groups—they either received no mammography screening, or they received a mammogram every two to three years. After only seven years, there has been a 31 percent reduction in deaths from breast cancer and a 25 percent reduction in advanced disease (*Lancet,* April 13, 1985).

"These results are truly exciting. They uniformly, and without question, demonstrate the effectiveness of mammography," Dr. Speroff says.

And these numbers should only get better with time. "As each year goes by, the women in the study get older, so more and more of them become at risk for breast cancer," Dr. Speroff explains. As more and more women in the unscreened group die of breast cancer, and fewer in the screened group die, mammography will prove just how much of a lifesaver it can be.

It doesn't take much figuring to see why mammography is so effective. It finds cancers long before they can be felt by hand, either by a woman or her doctor.

Most women, and doctors, can first detect a lump when it has grown to ⅝ inch in diameter. By this time, the cancer has been growing for eight to ten years. It has a 30 to 40 percent chance of having spread beyond the breast to the lymph nodes under the arm, and possibly to other parts of the body.

Mammography, on the other hand, can find lumps that are just half this size, or even smaller. The chances of the cancer having spread at this early stage are cut in half.

A mammogram can't tell you for sure if a lump is malignant or benign—only a microscopic study of cells from the mass can do that. And mammograms, unfortunately, cannot detect all cancers. Palpation remains necessary to detect the 10 to 15 percent that are not visible with mammography.

The American Cancer Society recommends a baseline mammographic screening for all women between ages 35 and 40 (this will be compared with future mammograms); a screening every one or two years for women ages 40 to 49, and annual screenings for all women age 50 and over.

Mammograms are seriously underutilized in this country. Most are done to confirm the presence of a lump found by palpation, not to find hidden lumps. It's estimated that less than half of women over age 50 have had a baseline mammogram, and that only 5 percent of women over age 50 have an annual mammogram.

It's time to ask your doctor if you should have mammography, Dr. Speroff suggests. "The true benefits of mammography have just become clear. Not every doctor is going to learn about this overnight." But they might learn about it a lot faster if their patients tip them off.

Exercise and Body Fat

Exercise may prove to be an unexpected ally in the fight against breast cancer, according to researchers at Harvard University. Their recent study was the first to show that long-term physical activity could protect against certain kinds of cancer (*British Journal of Cancer,* volume 52, 1985).

The researchers looked at 5,398 women who had graduated from ten U.S. colleges between 1925 and 1981. Half of the women had been college athletes—they'd trained at least twice a week for most of their college years at energy-intensive sports. Over 80 percent had begun their training by high school or earlier. The other half were nonathletes during this time.

"We found that the nonathletic women had almost twice the risk of breast cancer than did the former athletes," says Rose Frisch, Ph.D., a Harvard University School of Public Health professor and the study's director. The inactive women also reported about 2½ times as many cancers of the uterus, cervix, ovaries and vagina. The former college athletes were also found to have a lower risk of benign breast disease and benign tumors of the reproductive system.

The athletic women seemed to be particularly protected around the ages of 45 to 55, about the time of menopause. During this time, the risk for cancer of the reproductive organs and breasts normally rises rapidly. Among the nonathletes, the cancer rates rose in step with the general population. It also rose in the athletes, but much less.

"Exercise started early in life seems to have a long-range protective effect, as this finding illustrates," Dr. Frisch says.

To try to determine why this is so, researchers looked at a number of possible differences in risk factors between the groups—age, family history of cancer, age of first menstruation, number of pregnancies, use of birth-control pills or menopausal estrogen and smoking. They found that athletes and nonathletes did not differ much in many areas. It was true that many athletes did seem to have healthier lifestyle habits than their nonathlete counterparts—75 percent still exercise, for instance.

One marker in particular interested Dr. Frisch and colleagues—how fat the women were.

"I think that, in the long run, what may really make a difference is body composition—the amount of fat versus the amount of muscle you see on these women," Dr. Frisch says. "We think it's very likely that the former college athletes had been lean for a long time, although that was something we could not measure."

Body fat could be a vital link in the development of breast and other reproductive cancers, Dr. Frisch says. "We've known from other research for some time that fatter women make more estrogen and more potent forms of estrogen that have been related to increased cancers of the reproductive system. It's possible that the leaner women make less estrogen and less potent estrogen, and we hope to do research which clarifies this."

Women who begin exercising at a later age may still reap some protective benefits, Dr. Frisch believes. "We know cancer usually takes a long time to develop, and that highest risk is in the menopausal years. Women who begin exercising in their twenties or thirties have 25 years to get in good shape and stay that way."

Protective effects came with two to three hours a week of activity. "Some of the women in our exercise group who were at lower risk, for instance, ran two miles a day five days a week," Dr. Frisch says. "The exercise must be energy intensive and regular. But it doesn't have to be marathon running or Olympic training."

Breast Pain and Low-Fat Diets

Body fat, the amount of fat you eat, even the kinds of fat you eat—all seem related to certain breast ailments, including cancer. "They are all connected, although just how, we're not yet sure," says David Rose, M.D., Ph.D., D.Sc., chief of the American Health Foundation's division of nutrition and endocrinology.

In a preliminary study, Dr. Rose looked at the role of dietary fat in young women who had severe fibrocystic disease— painful, swollen lumpy breasts, especially premenstrually.

These women were instructed to eat a low-fat diet. Only 20 percent of their calories were to come from fat. "We found that they could do this, and we found that it worked," Dr. Rose says. After three months on the diet, all the women reported a reduction in breast pain. Not only that, but important hormones found in their blood had dropped dramatically. Blood levels of prolactin, a breast-stimulating hormone, and of two different forms of estrogen had all dropped by about a third. "We think the breast disease is caused by an overproduction of these hormones, which is influenced by dietary fat," Dr. Rose says.

Although these women did lose a little weight on this diet, they were not overweight to begin with. "Most were rather thin," Dr. Rose says. "So we don't think the slight weight loss produced the improvement. We think it was dietary changes." Dr. Rose is now involved in a second study to verify these encouraging results.

The National Cancer Institute has just begun two ten-year studies of 14,000 women to determine whether a low-fat diet retards recurrence of or prevents breast cancer. Both studies will involve a diet that limits fat to 20 percent or less of daily calories. One group will be women who have had two or more biopsies for breast disease or have a family history of cancer. The other group will be women who have already had cancer confined to the breast. The two studies may help confirm what past population studies suggest—that dietary fat is linked to cancer.

Fish Oils, Prostaglandins and Breast Cancer

There may be a kind of fat you'll want to eat if you're concerned about breast cancer. It's the polyunsaturated oil found in fish like mackerel, salmon, herring and tuna.

In experiments with mice and rats, done by Rutgers University professor Rashida Karmali, Ph.D., and others, fish oil was found to provide potent protection against breast cancer. "Fish oil inhibited the growth of transplanted tumors, blocked development of chemically induced tumors and lowered levels of a biochemical indicator of cancer activity," Dr. Karmali says.

She, and other researchers, believe the fish oils work in a very specific way. They affect the body's production of potent biochemicals known as prostaglandins, which may be involved in cancerous tissue growth.

"In the last eight to ten years, several investigators have shown very clearly that the products of a certain kind of fatty acid (arachidonic acid) are significantly increased in tumorous tissues," Dr. Karmali says. "We think this excessive prostaglandin formation may cause biologically important interactions in carcinogenesis. It may incite the formation of tumor cells, fostering tumor-cell proliferation. And we know that it leads to suppressed immune response."

Fish oils apparently lead to decreased prostaglandin production in a very direct way. They latch onto an enzyme that the prostaglandins need for production. The more of this enzyme the fish oils grab, the less remains available to be made into harmful prostaglandins.

Because of these findings, and because theories of how the fish oil works make sense, a study has just been started at Memorial Sloan–Kettering Cancer Center in New York City. Women with a family history of cancer, or who have had a biopsy showing precancerous changes, will be studied for the effects of fish oil on female hormone metabolism. "This research is very important to do," says principal investigator Michael Osborne, M.D. "The fish oil looks very interesting, but until we finish up our work, there is no evidence that it prevents cancer in humans. It's simply too early to say that."

Substituting salmon or mackerel for beef or pork might be your best bet for cancer protection, Dr. Karmali says. "That would cut back on overall fat intake while boosting dietary fish oil. We really have to look at the role of overall nutrition in breast-cancer prevention," she says.

The National Cancer Institute has recommended that you attempt to keep total dietary fat low. Some other studies have shown that a cut in fat to just 20 percent of calories may protect best against breast cancer. Studies have also revealed other dietary connections to breast cancer. Vitamins C, A, E and selenium all seem to play a protective role.

In a recent study by researchers at the Linus Pauling Institute, vitamin C delayed the development of breast cancer in mice bred to show a high incidence of breast tumors. In tissue cultures, vitamin A prevents the proliferation, or uncontrolled growth, of breast tissue cells.

Vitamin E and selenium, both potent antioxidants, seem to work even better as a duo. They may protect the breasts from harmful by-products of the breakdown of fats.

Check with your doctor if you're thinking of changing the kinds of food you eat or taking nutrient supplements as a guard against breast disease or breast cancer. It may be just what the doctor orders.

Cramping Out Is No Fun!

New York City Ballet dancer Patrick Hinson was in the middle of a pirouette-packed performance when, suddenly, his calf kinked out.

His show-must-go-on attitude kept Hinson on his toes. "I just kept telling myself, 'If you can get through this to a point where you can put your foot down flat, the cramp will go away.'" And that's just what happened, and not a moment too soon.

Most of us can sympathize with the agonized dancer. We've all had muscle cramps in the calf of a leg, the arch of a foot or just under the ribs. It's a few moments of intense, grabbing pain that then begins to ease off. Reach down to rub that recalcitrant calf and you can actually feel a knot or thickening in the lame leg. Severe cramps, like those that sometimes occur during convulsive seizures, can be so strong they snap bones. Even ordinary cramps frequently tear muscle tissue. That's why they so often leave a lingering ache.

Muscle cramps may seem to strike out of the blue, but that's only because their warning signals go unnoticed. If you're a frequent victim, you may be putting yourself into a position or situation where a cramp is unavoidable.

Compromising Position

Many cramps, and especially those that strike your legs at night, occur because your body has assumed a compromising position, says Israel Weiner, M.D., assistant professor of neurological surgery at the University of Maryland School of Medicine, Baltimore. Perhaps you've let your foot point downward, which automatically contracts the calf muscle somewhat. Then, consciously or unconsciously, you've tensed your calf muscle, contracting it still more. This position is the ideal setup for a cramp.

"When you contract the muscle, if there is nothing counteracting that movement, like another muscle or a tendon being stretched in opposition, the contracted muscle can shorten beyond its normal limit and go into an uncontrollable shortened state—in other words, a cramp," Dr. Weiner says. In bed, heavy or tucked-in blankets may push your feet down. Then, if you tense your leg muscles, as you inevitably do when you stretch or turn over, it's . . . *gotcha!*

Older people seem particularly prone to nighttime cramps, and are sometimes overtreated for this problem, Dr. Weiner says. "It's important for them to know that this problem is usually not serious, and that it can almost always be resolved without drugs." How? By loosening bed covers or using a board to keep the weight of the covers off your feet. If you sleep on your stomach, hang your feet over the edge of the bed. And keep your feet flexed upward toward your head when you're stretching your legs. That make the muscles on the front of your legs contract, providing opposition to the calf muscles.

High heels also throw the legs and feet into a cramp-prone position, as some fashion-conscious women have discovered. The plump and shapely calf is actually a contracted muscle. In fact, women who wear high heels constantly may so shorten their calf muscles that when they take the shoes off, they're unable to touch their heels to the ground. Their leg muscles act like they are constantly walking around on tiptoe, which is exactly what they are doing.

The Universal Antidote

Doctors, coaches and sufferers agree that the fastest, surest cure for a cramp is to stretch the affected muscles. If your calf cramps, for example, you can simply stand firmly on your flat foot and press down as hard as you can, or you can do more elaborate stretches. (See box on page 115.)

Cramps actually start when the nerves that control the muscles are prompted to misfire, for any number of reasons. Stretching, apparently, changes neural impulses, making the nerves change their signal from "contract" to "relax." Usually stretching relieves a cramp within seconds. And staying fit and limber can help prevent cramps.

Cramps that occur when you are active can be due to bad positioning, but they frequently have other causes, like an insufficient blood supply to the tissue, muscle fatigue or mineral depletion. When the cramp occurs can be the tip-off to what's causing the problem, says Mona Shangold, M.D., director of Georgetown University's Sports Gynecology Center and coauthor (with husband Gabe Mirkin, M.D.) of *The Complete Sports Medicine Book for Women* (Simon and Schuster, 1985).

What about Minerals?

"Cramps that occur when you first start to exercise are usually due to a mineral imbalance, such as a calcium, sodium or potassium deficiency or excess," Dr. Shangold says. "Abnormal blood levels of these minerals usually allow the muscle to contract but prevent it from relaxing."

The minerals work in fairly complex ways that are not entirely understood, says James Knochel, M.D., a researcher with the Veterans Administration Hospital in Dallas who has spent many years studying mineral-related muscular disorders.

"Mineral deficiencies can affect blood flow to muscles," Dr. Knochel says. "When you contract a muscle, for instance, it releases potassium into the surrounding tissue where it acts as a dilator of arteries in the muscle bed. This doesn't occur in someone who is potassium deficient. It's equivalent to putting a tourniquet around your arm and then attempting to use the arm, which produces a cramp." Perhaps that's one reason ballet dancer Patrick Hinson swears by potassium-packed bananas and baked potatoes.

A potassium deficiency also impairs the ability of the muscles to use glycogen, a sugar that is their main source of energy, Dr. Knochel says. This makes them weak and cramp-prone. Potassium and other mineral deficiencies may also affect the "excitability" of nerves—their tendency to fire off a series of muscle-cramping messages. And they may affect the muscles' "fatigue threshold"—their ability to do more work without becoming tired and spasm-prone.

Body mineral levels may be affected by hormonal changes or unusual physical demands. Pregnancy, too, can make women particularly prone to leg cramps.

In one recent study, researchers at Brigham Young University in Provo, Utah, found that 266 milligrams a day of supplemental magnesium reduced cramping in all their groups of pregnant women. The women were followed during the final two months of their pregnancy. The group with the most cramps—women over age 27 who already had at least one child—were helped the most by the magnesium. Their cramps were reduced by 57 percent.

Some clinical studies seem to indicate that additional calcium may reduce muscle cramps in pregnant women and growing children, who may be deficient in these minerals because of increased nutritional needs. Calcium and magnesium work closely together in the muscles, Dr. Knochel says.

While sodium deficiencies are another well-known cause of muscle cramps, most doctors no longer recommend salt tablets, since most people's diets already contain more than adequate salt. But, Dr. Knochel says, if you are a on a low-sodium diet and find you have muscle cramps, especially when you sweat heavily while working or exercising, too little salt may be your problem.

In any case, it's good to check with a doctor if you suspect a mineral deficiency is causing your muscle cramps. Mineral imbalances aren't particularly common, Dr. Shangold says. At risk are those taking diuretics or steroids, heavy drinkers, pregnant women and older people who may not be eating well.

Cramps that occur after you have exercised for a little while are most frequently caused by an inadequate blood supply to the muscle, Dr. Shangold says. "At rest, your arteries may be large enough to transport the small amount of blood that your muscles require to function properly. When you exercise, however, your muscles require large amounts of oxygen-rich blood. If your arteries are not large enough to transport enough blood, your muscles suffer from lack of oxygen and go into spasm."

What some older people mistake for a leg cramp is a condition known as intermittent claudication. It's a cramplike pain that comes on after a bit of exercise. It makes the leg feel heavy and weak.

Intermittent claudication is caused by clogged arteries in the leg, and its symptoms are similar to angina in the heart muscle, says Robert Layzer, M.D., professor of neurology at the University of California Medical Center at San Francisco. It's important to see a doctor if you have such symptoms, or any cramping pain in the legs accompanied by numbness or coldness in the affected leg or foot.

Most doctors recommend exercise, stopping smoking, a low-fat diet and drugs for this condition when it occurs in the lower leg. In some studies, vitamin E has also relieved symptoms, perhaps by reducing the tendency for red blood cells to clump together and form clots. In one study, supplementation with 600 international units (I.U.) of vitamin E daily for at least three months provided improvement for a number of patients. Those who got the vitamin E required far fewer leg amputations than those treated with placebos or other drugs. They were better able to walk. Blood circulation improved in their legs, although it sometimes took up to 25 months of supplementation before this result was apparent (*Vasa,* 2:280).

Dried-Up Muscles

Cramps that occur after you have been exercising for a long time are most often due to dehydration, Dr. Shangold says. "When you exercise for a long time, particularly in hot weather, you lose a lot of fluid. During a vigorous tennis match, for instance, a player can lose as much as two quarts of water per hour. Your blood volume is reduced, and there may not be enough blood to supply oxygen to all your exercising muscles. As a result, the most actively exercised muscles may not get enough blood, and they can go into spasm and hurt."

You can protect yourself from developing these kinds of cramps by drinking a glass of water before you exercise and at least every 15 minutes while you exercise, Dr. Shangold says.

Thorn in the Side

A stitch, or a side sticker, is a cramp in the diaphragm, the large muscle that separates your chest from your gut and controls breathing. The cramp occurs when this muscle doesn't get enough blood during exercise, Dr. Shangold says. "When you run, you lift your knees and contract your belly muscles, so that the pressure inside your belly increases and pushes on the diaphragm from below. At the same time, if you're breathing heavily you are expanding your lungs, which presses down on the diaphragm from above. This dual pressure squeezes the diaphragm and shuts off blood flow to it. The muscle can't get enough oxygen and goes into spasm."

If you develop a stitch, stop exercising, Dr. Shangold says. Push your fingers deep into your belly just below your ribs on the right side to stretch the diaphragm muscle with your hand. At the same time, purse your lips tightly and blow out as hard as you can. This should release the pressure on your diaphragm and stop the stitch.

It's true that if a swimmer gets an abdominal cramp, he may have trouble reaching shore safely. But contrary to popular belief, swimmer's cramps don't seem to depend on how recently you have eaten. They're more likely to be caused by fatigue or extreme exertion. "It's true that digesting food requires that some blood be shunted away from the heart and muscles," Dr. Shangold says. "But no healthy person should have trouble digesting food and swimming at the same time." In fact, the Red Cross no longer recommends that you wait for an hour after eating before you hit the surf.

No More Cramps

Preventive measures should keep most cramps at bay. But if an occasional one still sneaks up on you, try stretching it away with the simple exercises accompanying this article. Then, doctors say, if the area still hurts, treat it as you would an injured muscle, which is exactly what it is.

Rest the limb to avoid pain from further cramps or spasms and to keep from injuring the muscle even more. Apply ice to reduce swelling and pain.

Avoid getting a cramp in the first place by checking your body posture. Don't point your toes, or let your feet get pushed over by bedsheets. Don't set yourself up for a muscle injury, which may make you more susceptible to cramps. Train carefully. Avoid intense, jerky movements. Stretch to warm up and cool down. Don't bounce. Don't exercise beyond the point of fatigue. But do exercise. Sedentary people are prone to cramps, too. And see a doctor if you think a mineral deficiency may be your problem.

STRETCHES TO UNCRAMP YOUR LIFE

To stop or avoid a cramp, keep your muscles stretched and limber. These three stretching exercises are good for the calves and the arches of the feet, the muscles most likely to cramp.

1. Stand about three feet from a wall, or as far as you can, and keep your heels flat and legs straight. Point your feet straight ahead, lean into the wall, and rest on your hands and elbows. Hold 10 to 15 seconds, or longer if you can.

2. Sit on the floor with your leg straight, grab the top of your foot and pull forward. If your calf is cramped, Dr. Mona Shangold suggests that you also rhythmically squeeze the muscle. If you can't reach your foot with your hand, place a towel or belt around your foot and pull toward you.

3. Yoga poses provide an excellent way to stretch muscles. For calves and arms, try this position: Stoop on the floor, with feet flat, arms outstretched and hands flat on the floor in front of you. Slowly straighten your legs until your body forms the shape of a triangle, with your hips at the apex. Hold as long as it feels comfortable.

Ten Ways to Turn Back Cancer

Many of us have lived with a feeling of helplessness about cancer for so long that it's hard to change our thinking.

But a massive body of research now refutes the long-held belief that we are at the mercy of cancer, and instead shows that we can prevent it.

How much of an impact could we have if we all practiced prevention? "If it were possible that we could carry it out ideally, as much as 80 to 85 percent of all cancers today might not occur," says Charles A. LeMaistre, M.D., president of the American Cancer Society. "For too long we have regarded cancer as the dominant factor in its relationship with man. Now, preventing this disease is becoming more and more realistic."

By avoiding the things that are known to cause cancer, and incorporating into our lives factors that protect against it, we can reduce our risk of developing the disease.

"In some areas, the information is now so complete that it's unequivocal, such as the causal role of smoking in the development of cancer," says Dr. LeMaistre, who is also president of the University of Texas's M.D. Anderson Hospital and Tumor Institute, in Houston. "In other areas, such as diet and nutrition, information is not yet complete, but it is sufficient to take action."

The following ten steps summarize what we can do, and are recommended by the American Cancer Society. They will also contribute to a healthier life in general.

1. *Eat more high-fiber foods.* These include whole grains, fruits and vegetables. There is a lot of evidence that colon cancer is less common in populations that eat a diet high in fiber. In a study comparing Finnish and Danish people, for example, colon cancer was much lower among the Finns. The diets of the two groups are similar, except that the Finns eat large amounts of high-fiber, whole grain rye bread, while the Danes have a low-fiber diet.

Fiber may work by hastening the travel time of fecal matter through the bowel, so that carcinogens (cancer-causing substances) are whisked away before they can do their damage. Another theory is that by increasing the bulk of the stool, fiber dilutes the concentration of carcinogens.

2. *Eat more foods rich in vitamin A.* These include such things as spinach, carrots, sweet potatoes and apricots. It may help protect you against cancers of the lung, esophagus and larynx. In a major study, Norwegian men whose intake of vitamin A was above average had less than half the rate of lung cancer of men whose intake of the vitamin was below average.

Right now it's unclear whether the effects are due to vitamin A itself or a precursor of vitamin A called beta-carotene, a pigment found in plants. The emphasis now is on the naturally occurring pigment, because the precursors of vitamin A are the most probable agents that have this effect.

Beta-carotene is found in dark-green and deep-yellow vegetables, and in deep-yellow fruits.

3. *Get plenty of vitamin C.* Studies indicate that people whose diets are rich in vitamin C are less likely to get cancer, particularly of the stomach and esophagus.

We know that vitamin C can inhibit the formation of nitrosamines, cancer-causing chemicals, in the stomach. That may be how it protects against cancer.

Fruits and vegetables, particularly oranges, grapefruit, green peppers, broccoli, tomatoes and potatoes, are good sources of the vitamin.

4. *Eat more cabbage-family vegetables.* Such foods as broccoli, cauliflower, brussels spourts, cabbage, kale and kohlrabi fall in this category. Studies in large groups of people have suggested that consuming these vegetables, also called cruciferous vegetables, may reduce the risk of cancer, particularly of the gastrointestinal and respiratory tracts. And tests in laboratory animals reveal that cruciferous vegetables may be highly effective in preventing chemically induced cancer.

What is it about these foods that is protective? "We have to look upon these vegetables as a source of vitamins A and C and fiber, but there are other possibilities under investigation," Dr. LeMaistre told us.

5. *Trim fat from your diet.* Studies in humans and laboratory studies point out that excessive fat intake increases the chance of developing cancers of the breast, colon and prostate. And it's not just one kind of fat that's a problem—both saturated and unsaturated fats, whether of plant or animal origin, have been found to enhance cancer growth when eaten in excess.

The National Academy of Sciences recommends that we decrease the amount of fat in our diet to 30 percent of the total calories we eat (Americans currently consume about 40 percent of total calories as fat).

You can cut your fat intake by using less fats and oils in cooking, and by switching to lean meat, fish and low-fat dairy products.

6. *Control your weight.* "The long-standing and repeated observation that obesity is correlated with cancer is sufficiently substantiated to take action," says Dr. LeMaistre. In one mas-

UP-AND-COMING
CANCER PREVENTERS

The list of factors professed to prevent cancer is probably as long as the list of factors thought to promote it. With so many possibilities being bandied about, perhaps you've decided it's easiest to disregard the whole lot of them. But research does offer some promising leads worth pursuing.

Selenium, for example, is an essential trace mineral that reduces the occurrence of some cancers in animals. And statistics suggest a possible benefit in humans. In one study, researchers collected blood serum samples and stored them for up to five years. Selenium levels in people who later developed cancer were compared with levels in people free of cancer. The overall risk of cancer for those with selenium levels in the lowest fifth was twice that of people with levels in the highest fifth (*New England Journal of Medicine,* March 15, 1984).

Scientists speculate that selenium's antioxidant activity may be responsible for its protective effect. (Oxidation produces highly unstable molecules that are thought to initiate cancer.) But they also advise caution: Selenium is toxic in high doses.

Vitamin E, another antioxidant, is also being investigated as a possible preventer of cancer, especially of the breast. In a recent review of the available information, researchers cite evidence from laboratory and animal studies that vitamin E may decrease or inhibit tumor formation.

Two recent studies in humans had conflicting results, though. In the first, there was no correlation between serum vitamin E levels and breast cancer. In the second, there were five times as many breast cancer cases in women with low vitamin E levels. The researchers reviewing all the evidence think vitamin E is promising

sive study conducted by the American Cancer Society over 12 years, researchers found an increased incidence of cancers of the uterus, gallbladder, breast, colon, kidney and stomach in obese people. In that study, women and men who were 40 percent or more overweight had a 55 and 33 percent greater risk of cancer respectively than people of normal weight.

UP-AND-COMING
CANCER PREVENTERS— *Continued*

enough to recommend that large-scale clinical trials be carried out to find out for sure (*Journal of the American College of Nutrition,* vol. 4, no. 5).

Two newcomers among the cancer-prevention hopefuls are calcium and vitamin D. In a 20-year study by Cedric Garland, Dr. P.H., and colleagues at the University of California School of Medicine in San Diego, men who drank the least milk had almost three times the risk of getting colon or rectal cancer as those who drank the most (*Lancet,* February 9, 1985).

The researchers give the credit to calcium and vitamin D. They suspect that calcium combines with harmful bile acids and fatty acids in the intestine and escorts them safely from the body. They think that vitamin D may aid this function of calcium.

A very recent study provides more evidence of calcium's anticancer possibilities.

Researchers from Memorial Sloan-Kettering Cancer Center and Cornell University Medical College, in New York City, gave 1,250 milligrams of calcium a day (1.5 times the Recommended Dietary Allowance) to people from families that had increased frequencies of colon cancer. In people predisposed to colon cancer, an early sign is increased proliferation of cells lining the inside of the colon. Two to three months after supplementation was started, proliferation of these cells was significantly reduced in these people, and was almost the same as in people at low risk for colon cancer. In commenting on both studies, the researchers say ". . . high calcium intake is accompanied by both decreased cell proliferation in [cells lining the colon] and by a lower risk of colonic cancer" (*New England Journal of Medicine,* November 28, 1985).

Regular exercise and lower calorie intake can help you avoid gaining weight. It's advisable to check with your doctor before embarking on a special diet or strenuous exercise routine, though.

7. *Avoid salt-cured, smoked and nitrite-cured foods.* These include such foods as ham, bacon, hot dogs and salt-cured or smoked fish. Cancers of the esophagus and stomach are common in countries where large quantities of these foods are eaten.

Smoked foods absorb some of the tars from the smoke they're cured with. The tars contain cancer-causing chemicals similar to those in tobacco smoke. There is also good evidence that nitrate and nitrite can enhance the formation of nitrosamines in our food and in our digestive tract.

8. *Don't smoke cigarettes.* "About 30 percent of all cancer is clearly and unequivocally due to cigarette smoking," says Dr. LeMaistre. "It's been 20 years since the Surgeon General's Report on Smoking and Health, without any significant findings having been refuted." Smoking poses a risk to the nonsmoker (passive smoking) as well, he points out.

If you're a smoker and haven't quit because you think "the damage has already been done," take heart in the findings of a British study of over 18,000 people. Researchers found that people who had smoked for as long as 20 years—but who had been off cigarettes for 10 years or more—had no greater risk of lung cancer than people who had never smoked at all (*British Medical Journal*, June, 1984).

9. *Go easy on alcohol.* Heavy drinkers, especially those who also smoke, are at very high risk for cancers of the mouth and throat. Your risk of liver cancer also increases if you drink a lot.

10. *Shield yourself from the sun.* Too much sun causes skin cancer and other skin damage. "Like most other Americans, I'm learning that tanning of hide is neither healthy nor beautiful," says Dr. LeMaistre. "I use maximum-strength sunblocks and also use hats and other ways of shading myself."

A sunscreen with a Sun Protection Factor (SPF) of 15 or more gives maximum protection. Be especially wary during the midday hours—from 11:00 A.M. to 3:00 P.M.—when the sun is strongest. And don't use indoor sunlamps or tanning booths—they're not safe either.

Although they affect fewer people than the risk factors already mentioned, excessive x-rays, estrogens and exposure at work to harmful chemicals and fibers like asbestos should also be avoided. "I think every effort should be made to protect a human being from excessive x-rays and from the other known causes of cancer, albeit they cause a very small percentage of cancer today," says Dr. LeMaistre. You can ask your doctor about the need for x-rays and estrogens, and be familiar with proper safety procedures on the job.

Following all of the preventive steps may reduce your risk of cancer dramatically. But there's another side to cancer prevention—early detection. Sigmoidoscopy, Pap tests and breast exams, for example, can catch cancers when there's still a very good chance of curing them. For details on these and other lifesaving early-detection methods, contact your local American Cancer Society chapter or ask your doctor.

Allergy Defense Update

Robert Bricken of Owings Mills, Maryland, was pacing off part of his property when he trespassed on some particularly hazardous turf—a yellow jackets' nest. The insects took immediate offense, landing about 20 stings on Bricken's bare leg before he had a chance to retreat. Minutes later not only was his limb horribly swollen, but his face was beginning to puff up, too. "I looked in the mirror and couldn't recognize myself," Bricken recalls. "They say you sometimes have a sense of impending doom with this sort of reaction. Well, there for a while I wasn't sure what was going to happen to me."

Obviously, Bricken recovered, not only to tell his tale, but to gladly submit every few weeks to the allergy shots that protect him from further buzzing attacks. "I've been stung three times since, with no problems at all," he says.

It's true that few allergies are life threatening. More often, they simply disrupt life, making it impossible to keep a furry pet or stroll through an autumn woodland. Still, with 35 million suffering Americans, figuring out how allergies occur and the best ways to provide treatment are the goals of researchers around the country.

Immune System Gone Haywire

"An allergy is an abnormal reaction by the immune system to an ordinarily harmless substance," explains Charles H.

Banov, M.D., president of the American College of Allergists. "The immune system normally protects the body against harmful invaders, but in allergic people, it reacts to innocuous substances." The result is a long list of possible symptoms—wheezing, sneezing, swelling, itching, headache, nausea, fatigue, even deadly shock.

Researchers believe people who develop allergies have a genetic tendency to produce more than normal amounts of a type of antibody (or immunoglobulin) called IgE. This antibody acts as the link-up between allergy-producing particles of dust or pollen (called allergens or antigens) and the cells that produce the chemicals that cause the symptoms of allergy. The more IgE in the body, the stronger the allergic response.

Traditionally, allergists have followed a set course of evaluation and treatment: questions to determine the nature of your allergy; skin-prick or blood tests to pinpoint specific allergens; advice on what to avoid; or, if unavoidable, drugs to relieve symptoms or injections to desensitize. Updates in treatment basically have been refinements in these methods—better means of isolating allergens, new tests, purer injections and more effective symptom-suppressing drugs.

Isolating specific allergens in house dust, for example, lures some researchers. House-dust allergies have been particularly frustrating to treat. It's hard to avoid dust. And it's such a mixture of ingredients—molds, dander, wood dust and insects that change with the seasons—that it's been difficult to develop desensitizing shots that work well.

Many researchers think microscopic spiderlike animals called dust mites may be the worst allergy-producing substance in house dust. Found in humid, warm areas, dust mites settle on your rugs, bedding and furniture and feed off the gram or so of skin flakes you shed each week. There's no good way to get rid of them. "Both their droppings and body parts can cause asthma and nasal allergies," says Charles Reed, M.D., chairman of the Mayo Clinic's Allergy Division and an expert in house-dust allergies. Developing effective injections for dust-mite allergies can help solve the house-dust problem, Dr. Reed says. Until then, the current treatment is some fairly old advice—keep your house white-glove clean.

Testing for Allergies

Several tests are now available for diagnosing allergies. Not all of them work well. In the newest, RAST (short for radioallergosorbent test), a sample of a patient's blood is exposed to an allergen, then analyzed for allergy-producing IgE antibodies. The more antibodies, the stronger the allergic reaction. This test's advantage is that it requires a single blood sample. You don't have to endure a series of stabs.

But the RAST apparently has some problems. About 20 percent of its findings are false positives, indicating allergies for which you have no symptoms. That's why it's important to confirm RAST findings with a skin-prick test, says Anne Kagey-Sobotka, Ph.D., of the Johns Hopkins University School of Medicine, Division of Clinical Immunology. "The skin test is relatively painless, exquisitely sensitive and inexpensive," she says. "I don't think it will ever be replaced by the RAST."

Neither RAST nor skin tests are considered absolutely reliable for detecting food allergies. But they might be helpful under certain circumstances, Dr. Banov says. And cytotoxic testing, a method used by some allergists to detect food allergies, is considered unproven and unreliable, according to a recent Food and Drug Administration report. The tests show many false positives, and don't correlate well with apparent symptoms.

"There's no question that food allergies do exist, and that we have a lot more to learn about them," Dr. Banov says. "The problem has been that it's very easy to incorrectly associate symptoms with foods. Food allergies often have been overdiagnosed."

When true food allergies exist, they often produce a detectable allergic reaction or immunological response, just as hay fever or stinging insect reactions do, Dr. Banov says. Most likely to produce this response are eggs and milk, especially in young children; chocolate, nuts, shellfish and tomatoes. Symptoms may include mild nausea, headaches, skin rash, hives, severe asthma or shock.

But some people have similar symptoms without the antigen-antibody reaction. "They are intolerant of a substance such as a food or drug, but they don't have what we think of as an allergy," Dr. Banov says. "A good example of this might be a medication that can produce asthma, congestion, polyps and hives in certain sensitive individuals, but not through an antigen-antibody reaction. People are not allergic to that substance, but they can be intolerant."

For diagnosing both allergies and intolerances to foods, "There is no question that the best way is an elimination diet, eating for a while only foods you know for sure are not causing your symptoms, then challenging your body by eating what you think is a problem food," he says.

Once the offender is identified, the advice is clear: "Shots for food allergies are completely ineffective," Dr. Banov says. "There is no way to treat a food allergy except to avoid the food."

Allergic to Modern Life?

Some people claim to have allergic reactions to pollutants, food chemicals or other substances in the environment— chlorinated water, natural gas, synthetic fibers, cigarette smoke, soap powder, perfume, exhaust fumes. Some doctors isolate the patient for several days in a nonallergic room, then, one by one, expose them to substances and observe for reactions.

"There are many false reactions because of the power of suggestion and emotional factors," he says. "Many patients find it easier to accept an allergy as the basis of their problems.

"It's true that certain substances can produce allergic reactions in some people," Dr. Banov says. "But most of these substances are irritants, or triggers, not true allergens. The antigen-antibody reaction is not present, although exposure to these irritants can cause a reaction in the allergy-prone person." The same advice follows, though, whether it's a trigger or a true allergen. Try to avoid symptom-causing substances.

Immunotherapy, or desensitizing injections, is appropriate when allergy symptoms are year-round and can't be avoided and when symptoms are dangerous or particularly annoying, Dr. Banov says. The shots work best for ragweed, grasses, certain tree pollens, molds and stinging insects. They don't work as well for dust or pets.

In immunotherapy, the doctor gives extracts of an allergen in gradually increasing dosages. This makes the body produce more of a certain kind of "blocking" antibody (called IgG), which can react with the allergy-producing particle before it reaches cells. In time, the patient acquires some protection against the allergen, just as he would after being vaccinated for an infection.

Usually, injections are given once or twice a week and are gradually reduced to once a month, ending after up to three years or sometimes longer. But a new form of allergy extract currently up for FDA approval may speed the immunizing process.

Researchers at Johns Hopkins University School of Medicine have been able to modify some antigens in ways that make it possible to desensitize a patient with about half the usual number of shots. "Our shots are less allergenic. That is, they are less likely to trigger a serious reaction than standard extracts," says Dr. Kagey-Sobotka. "But they have the equal ability to cause a protective IgG buildup." At the Johns Hopkins Allergy Clinic, these shots are available for allergies to ragweed and grasses. "We expect they will soon be available for other allergies, too," Dr. Kagey-Sobotka says.

Allergies to cats, dogs or birds can be particularly disheartening. In most people, they may ot appear until several years after initial contact with a pet, by which time emotional attachment could be strong.

"Although most allergists tell their patients to get rid of their pets, they know that about half these people will endure their symptoms rather than part with a beloved animal," says John Ohman, M.D. Dr. Ohman heads the Boston Veterans Administration outpatient allergy clinic and is a professor and researcher in pet allergies at Tufts University School of Medicine.

Injections to desensitize for animal allergies may not always be particularly effective, Dr. Ohman says. That's why most allergists don't like to use them unless a person simply can't avoid contact.

"I've given them to veterinarians, animal laboratory workers and social workers and police officers who have to visit houses where there could be pets," he says. In rare instances he's also given them to people who are so strongly attached to their pets they would rather endure the regimen of shots than life without Fido. "Some doctors are quite willing to do this," he says. "Other are very hesitant."

Several years ago, Dr. Ohman's research group developed a highly purified allergy injection that was very effective in reducing wheezing, sneezing and watery eyes in people allergic to cats. The injections contained a protein found in cat saliva. Unfortunately, this purified form of the allergen is not currently available to the public. "It's being worked on," Dr. Ohman says. "I would hope something like this will be available before too long."

Are You Really Protected?

Until recently, the only way a doctor could confirm that his patient was desensitized was by exposing him to an allergen and hoping for the best. In some cases, that exposure could be dangerous if the shots hadn't been effective. Now, though, blood tests that measure IgG blocking antibodies can be used to confirm desensitization in stinging insect, ragweed and grass allergies, and should be available soon for other kinds of allergies. (There's a similar test to determine one's reactivity to penicillin.)

"In the 1,000 or so patients we've studied, we have found what we feel is a protective level of IgG," Dr. Kagey-Sobotka says. "A person who has more than 4 micrograms of IgG in his blood is essentially at no risk from a sting, even if he has had a catastrophic reaction before. We give him immunotherapy for a few weeks, check his blood IgG levels, and continue immunotherapy until IgG reaches a protective level. If we're worried about whether a patient is responding or whether we need to increase the dosage, we check the IgG level."

Many people who have severe reactions to insect stings apparently have been stung previously with no reaction, Dr. Kagey-Sobotka says. "Symptoms indicating you should look into shots include difficulty breathing, dizziness and swelling of the throat and face. Bad swelling at the site of the sting, though, seems not to portend a later life-threatening reaction."

Drugs to Relieve Symptoms

A number of drugs can relieve allergy symptoms and often that is all that is needed. In many cases drugs are given along with allergy shots.

Antihistamines are most commonly used. These drugs block the action of histamine and other related chemicals that can contract air passages or cause sneezing or itching. They are especially useful for treating hives and hay fever. Some people take antihistamines for years with good results, Dr. Banov says.

Many people complain that antihistamines make them drowsy. However, a new kind of antihistamine recently approved by the FDA does not cause drowsiness because it does not travel to the brain. The drug, chemically known as terfenadine, is available only by prescription. "It can have side effects of causing dryness, prostate retention in males, visual difficulties and in rare cases, sedative effects," says Dr. Banov. "But it has many fewer side effects than standard antihistamines."

Cells that release histamine also cause the release of other powerful chemicals, and researchers are looking for ways to block their effects, too. One recently identified group of biochemicals, known as leukotrienes, may have even more potent effects than histamine, says Dr. Kagey-Sobotka. "We think leukotrienes play an important part in asthma and other breathing problems. They cause constriction and loss of elasticity in tiny air passages in the lungs, which can seriously hinder the passage of oxygen into blood."

Researchers around the country are working to find drugs that block the actions of leukotrienes and the other biochemicals involved in allergic response, Dr. Kagey-Sobotka says. When they do, it will be a major breakthrough in allergy treatment. "And there's no doubt that these drugs will be developed. It's only a matter of time."

Are Food Allergies Feeding Your Health Problem?

You're not alone if you're convinced there are some foods you're better off leaving on your plate. Perhaps you've noticed a stomach upset, headache or rash after you've eaten a certain food. And maybe you've discovered you feel better when you avoid that food for a few days. You may even have had tests to try to pinpoint the foods causing your symptoms.

If you've found the help you need, you are lucky. Traditionally, most allergists have disregarded food-related symptoms, while the typical food-allergy specialist has been considered something of a quack. It certainly hasn't helped that a commonly used means of food-allergy diagnosis, cytotoxic testing, has been found unreliable; or, that some reactions dubbed "allergy" are delayed responses that don't show up on standard allergy tests. The problem, for doctors traditional or otherwise, has been a lack of good, solid research. That's why the newest studies in this field are so exciting. In the past, most studies of food sensitivity or allergy hadn't followed standard scientific protocol. As a result, their findings were ignored by the medical community.

Now these findings are being looked at anew, this time by top researchers in allergy and immunology, who are conducting carefully controlled studies. This is research that will, finally, begin to separate fact from fiction. It promises to give the study of food-related ailments a credibility and acceptance it has so far lacked and to provide details of biochemistry that were previously speculative. The following studies are some of the first to do this.

That certain foods can cause migraine headaches is well accepted, although how so is still being determined. Symptoms triggered by red wine, aged cheeses or herring are apparently due to a metabolic disorder, says Lyndon Mansfield, M.D., chief of immunology/allergy at Texas Tech University Health Sciences Center, in El Paso. Other foods or additives work like chemicals or drugs in sensitive people. These include caffeine, alcohol, monosodium glutamate and nitrates.

But some migraineurs apparently have a true allergic reaction to often-eaten foods like wheat, milk, eggs, corn and sometimes peanuts.

In Dr. Mansfield's study, 43 migraine sufferers were given skin-prick tests for allergies to 83 foods. The 16 people with positive results eliminated those foods from their diet for a month. Those whose skin tests were negative went one month without milk, egg, corn or wheat. All recorded their diets, headaches and medicine use in a daily diary.

On the elimination diet, 13 patients improved, 11 from the skin-positive but only two from the skin-negative group. The people whose symptoms improved had only about one-third the number of headaches they'd had before going on the diet.

Seven of those who improved agreed to undergo a double-blind placebo-controlled oral challenge. In this kind of test, foods are dried and hidden in either capsules or a mash. Neither the researcher giving nor the volunteer eating the food knows whether it's thought to be allergenic or not. This way, the volunteer will not have a psychosomatic reaction to a food he considers allergenic, and researchers will be unable to unconsciously show their own bias.

In five of these volunteers, food allergy was confirmed. In three who allowed blood samples to be taken during the food challenge, researchers measured levels of histamine, an important biochemical marker of allergic reaction. In all of the volunteers, histamine levels rose.

"Measuring histamine, a blood-vessel dilator, is an important first step in determining the mechanism by which some foods can cause allergic migraines," Dr. Mansfield says.

Early researchers in food allergy believed the most reactive foods were those people ate most often. "And in fact, it looks like they were right," Dr. Mansfield says. "Wheat was a common migraine trigger, and has since come up in a number of people not in our report."

Like many other researchers in this field, Dr. Mansfield is a former skeptic. "I thought people involved in this field were way off base in their ideas. Now I believe food is a real provoker in certain cases. Six of the people in my study had no headaches staying on their elimination diet, and that's much better than having to take a lot of medicine" (*Annals of Allergy,* August, 1985).

The Case for Irritable Bowel

Several studies in the last few years indicate food sensitivities may play a role in irritable-bowel syndrome, where diarrhea or constipation, pain and gas play havoc with one's innards. In fact, researchers at Cambridge University's department of immunology found that two out of every three irritable bowel sufferers in their study remained symptomless when they followed an elimination diet.

The British researchers found that foods provoked symptoms in 14 of 21 patients with irritable bowel. In 6, a double-blind challenge confirmed the intolerance. Wheat, corn, dairy products, coffee, tea and citrus fruits were the most likely offenders.

All patients found to be intolerant of wheat had an intestinal biopsy; in all, samples were normal. There were no signs of *celiac,* a wheat-intolerance disease, or of *Crohn's,* an inflammatory disease that causes scarring and thickening of the bowel wall.

And while many people who react to dairy products lack a digestive enzyme that breaks down milk sugars, not all do. Some may have a food intolerance. When they eat a dairy product, the colon produces large amounts of prostaglandins, biochemicals that might contribute to diarrhea.

Irritable-bowel syndrome has often been considered a psychosomatic reaction to stress. The British researchers leave no doubt, though, that doctors might be negligent to assign the symptoms to stress alone.

"Although stress undoubtedly exacerbates irritable bowel in some cases and other factors may be relevant, food intolerance appears to be very important in the diagnosis of this condition," the researchers write. It takes determination and understanding to come up with a diet to relieve symptoms, they note. "However, the benefits justify the effort required by patient, dietitian and doctor." And follow-up studies show that former irritable-bowel sufferers who stick with their elimination diets maintain their improvement.

When he first decided to look at the role diet might play in atopic dermatitis, an itchy, eczemalike skin disease, Hugh Sampson, M.D., of Duke University's School of Medicine, also was skeptical, with good reason. Many of the children in his study had tried various elimination diets, without much success.

But he found that 52 percent of the children had an allergic response to one or more foods. They reacted with scratching and redness within 15 to 90 minutes of eating. Some also experienced another response up to eight hours later. Quite a few children had not just rashes, but nausea or diarrhea, and a smaller number, wheezing or severe nasal congestion.

Six foods accounted for more than 85 percent of the positive responses. Eggs produced nearly half the reactions, followed by peanuts, milk, soy, wheat and fish. Although most of the children had positive skin-prick tests to several foods, most who reacted to the oral challenge did so to only one or two foods. That's why the oral challenge is so important in diagnosing an active food allergy, according to Dr. Sampson. It's the only accurate way to see if you truly have an allergic reaction.

"Some doctors recommend diets based only on skin-test results," Dr. Sampson says. "This has often meant that people have been put on a more restrictive diet than is necessary to control their symptoms, with up to 12 or more foods eliminated. So either the parents attempt to comply and the child is on a nutritionally deficient diet, or they throw up their hands and say, 'No way. We can't do it.' " Those are two reasons the elimination diets these children were on earlier failed.

"With the food challenge, we have found most children only react to one or two foods. They can eat everything but those foods."

Parents, and Dr. Sampson, have seen significant improvements in the children who stuck to the allergy-free diet compared to those not treated for allergy.

And when they were checked for allergy again a year or two later, 40 percent had lost their hypersensitivity. That's not surprising, Dr. Sampson says. As a child matures, he usually reacts to fewer foods, because the cells lining his intestines become less permeable to food allergens. That's also why there seem to be many more food sensitivities in children than in adults, he says, "although the incidence in adults remains largely unknown and should be studied" (*Journal of Pediatrics,* November, 1985).

W. T. Kniker, M.D., chief of the division of clinical immunology, department of pediatrics at the University of Texas Health Sciences Center, San Antonio, also studied eczema but in a group of children and adults whose allergic status was not known. He found that 75 percent of the children and more than 40 percent of the adults in his study improved when they went on a nonallergic diet and all began to have symptoms again when certain foods were returned to their diet. Half of these reacted within two hours and tended to show positive skin-prick-test responses. But the other half reacted more slowly, and even though their food challenge was clearly positive they did not have positive skin-prick-test responses. Most showed sensitivities to milk, soy, eggs, peanuts, chocolate and wheat. Keeping away from the protein foods continued the improvement of these patients.

A controversial area of research has been the relationship between food intolerance and mental symptoms. For years, researchers have observed anxiety, depression, irritability and hyperactivity in some people after they've eaten certain foods. Only recently, though, have controlled studies begun to clarify these observations. Recommending a food-additive-free diet for hyperactive children may be helpful for some children. At least, that's the conclusion reached by British researcher Joseph Egger, M.D., and his associates at the prestigious Hospital for Sick Children in London (*Lancet,* March 9, 1985).

Using an elimination diet followed by double-blind food challenges, Dr. Egger found that tartrazine (yellow dye No. 5) and the preservative benzoic acid caused hyperactive behavior in more than 70 percent of the children who initially improved on an elimination diet. (In the United States, both these substances must be listed on the labels of foods and drugs.)

He also found that about 25 percent of the children reacted to milk, soy, chocolate, peanuts, grapes, wheat, oranges, eggs, corn, fish or oats. While many of the other children did have other symptoms of allergy, skin-prick testing was unreliable in predicting who would respond to food challenge.

"This trial indicates that the suggestion that diet may contribute to behavior must be taken seriously," Dr. Egger says.

Anxiety, Depression in Adults

Apparently it's not just children who may experience behavior changes from food triggers. Some adults seem to react, too, according to research at the University of Chicago Medical Center.

"Such a link has long been theorized but has seldom been studied and almost never shown," says study director John Crayton, M.D. "We wanted to know if this could be demonstrated under strictly controlled conditions and to explore the mechanisms that might be at play."

The study involved 23 psychiatric patients with a history of food-reaction complaints and 12 normal people with no such history.

The participants were placed on an eight-day program of double-blind food challenges of wheat, milk, chocolate or placebo. During that time, they underwent behavioral, mood assessment and other neuropsychological tests four times a day, and blood chemistry and immune-system analyses twice every day.

"Only one of the normal subjects appeared to react to a food, while 16 of the 23 people who complained in the past of food sensitivity showed significant mood and behavior changes during the study," Dr. Crayton said. Wheat or milk was linked to irritability, anxiety and depression. "Depression was very common, and was usually delayed some hours. It seemed as though the depths of the depression frequently occurred the next day," Dr. Crayton said. Chocolate was less likely to be connected with such mood effects.

One criticism of food-mood studies is that people who become sick from a food will naturally feel irritable or depressed. In this study, people reporting physical reactions like upset

WHAT'S AN ELIMINATION DIET?

The premise of an elimination diet and food challenge is simple enough.

First, stop eating all the foods you think might be causing your allergy symptoms. Then, when you are symptom-free, add foods back one by one, and note which cause symptoms to reappear.

There are several ways to come up with the initial allergy-free diet. Some doctors fast their patients on spring water for a few days. Others use a nonallergic, predigested liquid food like Vivonex. Neither should be done without medical supervision. Most, though, put their patients on a limited diet of foods generally considered nonallergic, says Richard Podell, M.D., a New Providence, New Jersey, internist and allergist. It may include lamb, rice, pears, water, salt, green beans, sweet potatoes and a cooking oil.

Dr. Podell, who is a clinical associate professor at the University of Medicine and Dentistry of New Jersey-Rutgers Medical School, keeps patients on this diet up to three weeks. "If they do not improve during this time, then food is probably not their problem," he says. "If they do improve, and many do, then you add new foods one at a time, and see which trigger their symptoms."

In a research setting, Dr. Podell says, it is important to do this double-blind, with a placebo. "But in clinical practice, that's time-consuming and cumbersome. So most doctors do it openly. We usually introduce each food back in three successive meals. And if they seem to react adversely, we put that food on our suspect list. We then go back and verify those foods with a second challenge. Usually, we can figure out which foods are really important to avoid, which can sometimes cause symptoms, and which are safe to eat all the time."

stomach were eliminated. And any physical complaints the remaining patients had were accounted for in their psychological rating. The food reactors also showed marked changes in two immune-system components when compared with the controls. Their blood showed significantly lower levels of a group of proteins that control immune-system response and higher levels of proteins formed as a result of allergic response. "Both these components are known to be related to a variety of illnesses that can affect various body systems, including, it seems, the brain," Dr. Crayton says.

How many people might have mood problems related to foods? That's not yet known, Dr. Crayton says. "If you think you're a reactor, I suggest you keep a diary to see if there is a relationship between what you are eating and how you feel."

Dr. Crayton did find that vulnerable people tended to crave or eat very frequently the foods to which they responded, something earlier researchers also noted. He and other researchers have also found that when an allergic food is first withdrawn, symptoms worsen for a day or two, then gradually improve.

The initial increase in symptoms is almost like a period of "drug withdrawal," and may drive someone to compulsively eat the food.

Like others in his field, Dr. Crayton is excited about the possibilities offered by further research. "It may mean that people with significant illnesses can improve simply by avoiding certain foods," he says.

Dr. Mansfield echoes those thoughts. "If you think you have a food allergy, it's definitely worth having it checked out."

Put Youth Back in Your Spine!

Can you get out of a car in one seamless motion? Work in your garden without wondering how you are going to straighten up at the end of the day? Make love with no fear that your body is going to kink up in some weird position that only an emergency medical team can undo?

You can if your spine is strong and flexible, able to bounce back from the stress of daily life. If it isn't that way with you, you can at least move in that direction by revitalizing the muscles, bone, cartilage and nerves that make up your spine. How? With a program of careful exercise, nutrition and lifestyle changes. Here's how to get started.

Join an Exercise Class for People with Back Problems and Stick with It ● Even many surgeons who used to pooh-pooh its benefits now agree exercise can be your spine's salvation.

"Most back pains written off as disk problems are really muscle problems," says Willibald Nagler, M.D., New York Hospital/Cornell University Medical Center's physiatrist-in-chief. (A physiatrist is an M.D. specializing in physical medicine and rehabilitation.) "Most people with back problems have back and hamstring muscles too tight for toe touching, and abdominal muscles too weak for sit-ups."

The back and hamstring muscles support the entire structure of the back. They must be strong but flexible, to enable you to bend over, sit or twist without straining your back.

The abdominal muscles, when strong, help to stabilize the lower back, the spine's most vulnerable point. Weak stomach muscles allow an exaggerated curve in the lower back, a posture that crimps disks and nerves.

To stretch the back and hamstring muscles, Dr. Nagler prescribes a series of exercises, including knee-to-chest pulls, cat curls and hip rolls. To tighten the stomach, he recommends half sit-ups with knees bent, alternate leg lifts, pelvic tilts and other exercises.

An excellent program incorporating many of these exercises is "The Y's Way to a Healthy Back," offered at most YMCAs. One word of warning: Rest, not exercise, is best when you are in true pain. And no exercise should hurt your back.

Assume the "S" Stance ● The trick to standing, and walking, is to find a posture that feels comfortable but offers your back maximum support. "We want to maintain the gentle 'S' curve of the spine," says Terry Nordstrom, director of the department of physical and occupational therapy and originator of the Back School of Stanford University. For some, in the case of the swayback, it helps to pull in the stomach and tuck under the buttocks. This tilts the pelvis toward the back and provides crucial support for the lower spine. Keep your knees slightly flexed, too.

When you're standing a long time, you can tilt the pelvis

back and flatten the small of your back by placing one foot on a stool, chair railing or other object a few inches high.

Sit Pretty ● Here again, you want to maintain the back's "S" curve. "People with lower back pain tend to flop into a chair or sofa, throwing their backs into a drooping 'C' shape," says Edgar Wilson, M.D., a University of Colorado professor with a special interest in psycho-physiology. This posture overstretches the lower back ligaments, while compressing the nerves passing out of the spinal column.

The easiest way to avoid slouching is to use a small pillow two or three inches thick behind your lower back when you sit. And avoid prolonged sitting. Take a stand-up break every hour.

Invest in a Good Chair ● Choose a chair that helps you to sit comfortably erect, not slumped forward. The ideal chair has a tiltable back support and adjustment height so you can sit with your feet flat on the floor and knees slightly lower or level with your hips.

It has a contoured seat pan, not a square cushion, to help equalize pressure on the underside of your thighs, and armrests to reduce stress getting in and out of the chair.

Don't Drive Yourself Crazy ● If you're shopping for a new car, look for seats that offer good back support. Today many manufacturers are aware of the selling qualities of comfortable, supportive seating. Equip your older car with an orthopedic form. Keep the seat forward so your knees are raised to hip level; your right leg should not be fully extended.

Give Your Spine the Nourishment It Needs ● Osteoporosis and arthritis add to the back problems of many older people, especially women. Back pain can be a sign of microscopic fractures in the vertebrae, as the spine slowly crumbles from age-related calcium losses. Many bone specialists today agree that, to prevent osteoporosis, most women should be getting at least 1,000 milligrams of calcium a day. That's about twice the current intake.

Vitamin D helps you absorb and use calcium. In one study, added vitamin D compound (calcitriol) reduced fractures in older women by 80 percent. If you're not drinking vitamin D-fortified milk or spending at least 15 minutes a day in the sun, consider taking a 400 international unit vitamin D supplement daily.

Trace minerals like zinc, copper and manganese are also vital to bone maintenance.

Include shellfish, liver, nuts, seeds and whole grains in your diet to help meet these requirements.

Some researchers suggest vitamin C could help maintain spinal disks, because it helps form collagen, a tough connective tissue covering disks. Others have found that B complex also helps maintain bone and cartilage as well as soothe nerves irritated by rubbing vertebrae. And some doctors use supplemental magnesium to help relieve the muscle spasms that can cause acute back pain.

Check Your Footgear ● Any kind of pounding your feet take can show up as back pain, especially if your muscles are weak (strong muscles are good shock absorbers) or you're older (aging spinal disks become thin and hard, providing less cushioning for vertebrae).

Switching to flexible-soled shoes with soft, shock-absorbing cushions produced significant pain relief in many patients treated in the orthopedics department of an Israeli hospital. The cushioning shoe inserts reduced—by 42 percent—incoming "shock waves" from pounding feet.

Avoid heels higher than 1¾ inches, which shift body weight forward and exaggerate swayback.

Visit a Back Store ● All kinds of goodies to pamper your back, including specially designed furniture and tools, positioning pillows, books and traction devices, can be found in a new kind of specialty shop—the back store. Check the phone book of the biggest city near you.

Learn to Lift ● Never bend over from the waist, even to pick up light objects, Nordstrom says. Bending from the waist deprives your spine of the support of the back muscles, which must relax to allow your body to flex. This places abnormal and uneven pressures on spinal disks. Squat close to the object, instead, bending at the knees with your back straight and stomach muscles tensed. Then, stand up slowly, holding heavy objects close to your body.

Clean Out Your Pocketbook ● An overweight pocketbook can do a number on your back, Nordstrom says. "We tell people to clean out their purses and briefcases, and to carry them as close to the body as possible. Over-the-shoulder is better than by hand." Try to keep your body from tilting in response to the weight of the object. And frequently switch the bag to the other shoulder. A backpack is a good alternative to the shoulder bag.

Drop Your Guard ● Relaxed muscles are less likely to go into painful spasms. "People who have been in pain for a while tend to tighten their muscles to guard the area, which makes it almost like a block of concrete," says Dr. Wilson.

Gentle stretching exercises, like yoga, are a good way to relax muscles. Biofeedback and progressive relaxation training can help you relax deeply, even while you're active.

Muscle-relaxing pills relieve acute back spasms, but, says Dr. Wilson, "I think they're terrible for long-term use. They completely separate a person from any awareness of his body. And that just makes things worse. Anti-inflammatory drugs such as aspirin or ibuprofen are helpful during the acute phase of back pain."

Walk like a Rag Doll ● People with bad backs tend to walk ramrod stiff, Dr. Wilson says. "We have them walk as they imagine a Raggedy Ann doll would—floppy and leaning forward slightly, with knees slightly flexed, exaggerating the bouncy, relaxed walk we want them to develop."

Find Your Painless Position ● "The key for anyone in acute pain is to rest in a neutral, supportive position," says Nordstrom.

"You can lie on your back with several pillows under your

legs and your knees somewhat bent. That reduces the stress on your back quite a bit and is usually most comfortable," Nordstrom says.

"If you lie on your side, put a pillow or small roll under your waist and a pillow between your legs. If your like lying on your stomach, put pillows under your belly to support your lower back."

Don't Take It Lying Down ● The old recommendation that a firm bed is best for a bad back is being revised. Too many people with aches and pains found that hard mattresses made them hurt more. Today, back experts recommend instead a bed that is level, with no sags, and firm enough to fully support the lower back.

"One suggestion I've found most helpful is to get a sheepskin or a soft inch-thick foam cover for their hard mattress," says Maggie Lettvin, former Massachusetts Institute of Technology fitness lecturer and author of *Maggie's Back Book* (Houghton-Mifflin).

Sleep like a Baby ● "Sleeping positions make a big difference," Lettvin says. Instead of lying on your back or stomach, she recommends sleeping in a fetal position—on your side with your knees bent at a right angle to your body, with small pillows under your waist and between your knees if needed.

Seek the Heat ● A warm bath or heating pad helps muscles relax. If you find yourself hunched into your blankets in the morning, wear a turtleneck shirt to bed, Dr. Wilson suggests.

When it's cold outdoors, keep your lower back warm with a jacket that covers your buttocks.

Lose That Excess Baggage ● Fat and back pain are an inseparable couple. "Especially when that weight is around their waist, people are likely to have back problems," Nordstrom says. The weight greatly stresses soft back tissues and compresses disks.

For maximum back protection and surest weight loss, combine diet with exercise.

Enroll in a Back School ● Some hospitals, university medical centers and private physical-therapy clinics offer programs where you learn how to exercise, sit, stand, work and play in ways that help, rather than hurt, your back. Ask at the physical-therapy department of a local hospital for the location of the back school nearest you.

How's That . . . Hearing of Yours?

The crowd dances while multicolored lights flash and music reverberates through Manhattan's trendiest new disco.

Hundreds of miles away, as the last light of day fades across the fields, a farmer turns his tractor toward home. Meanwhile, a young lawyer in San Francisco finishes tying his jogging shoes, snaps his small earphones into place, and heads for a run in Golden Gate Park.

In spite of their different situations, what do all these people have in common? They are all engaged in activities that could cause permanent hearing loss.

"If you happen to be a particularly sensitive individual, you may permanently lose part of your hearing if you're exposed to high-intensity sound at a close range," says Maxwell Abramson, M.D., professor and chairman of the department of otolaryngology at Columbia University's School of Medicine in New York City.

Loud disco music, noisy tractors and earphones turned up full volume are examples of the high-intensity sound Dr. Abramson is talking about.

Some noise merely annoys, Dr. Abramson points out, without actually damaging the ear.

"There may be psychological effects brought on by noise in the 90-decibel range but there won't be permanent hearing loss. Noisy restaurants, for example, may be annoying but they won't damage your ears."

How much noise is too much? Short of always taking along a gadget that gives a computer readout of surrounding decibel levels, understanding the ways in which noise can be harmful is the first step in maintaining healthy hearing. There are three factors that determine whether a specific sound might be damaging, Dr. Abramson explains: the intensity of the sound (how loud it is), its duration and its impulse quality.

An extremely loud noise produces sound waves that rush through the ear with such force that parts of the cochlea—the coiled tube in the inner ear—might be damaged. In the cochlea are thousands of tiny hairs that pick up vibrations from sound waves, transferring them along the auditory nerve to the brain. When they are blasted by excessively powerful sound waves, some of these little hairs may be torn away from their supporting structure, like trees ripped out in a tornado. Although healing sometimes occurs, if the damage is too severe, permanent hearing loss may result.

Occasional short bursts of loud sound are less apt to cause permanent damage than continuous exposure over long periods of time. In an effort to establish guidelines that will help protect people whose work exposes them to continuous loud noise, U.S. Department of Labor regulations list noise levels to which workers can be exposed without sustaining appreciable hearing loss. For example, a worker can be exposed to a maximum of 90 decibels for 8 hours a day, 92 decibels for 6 hours and 95 decibels for 4 hours. Exposure to these sound levels for greater lengths of time may result in hearing loss.

While even the healthiest ears risk being damaged by high volume and long exposure, someone whose ear may have been previously injured is even more vulnerable to future hearing loss, according to Dr. Abramson. "If there is pre-existing inner-ear damage, you will be more susceptible to noise injury," he warns.

Music That Hurts

Eight hours a day at a noisy job may be one thing, but surely an evening in a loud disco or at a rock concert can't really damage the ears—or can it?

"The loudest rock concerts can reach 110 decibels, maybe even more right up on stage where the musicians are," warns Robert Cubbage, a recording engineer in Manhattan.

If you have trouble grasping the concept of just how loud 110 decibels is, think of it this way: It's louder than the sound you would hear standing 50 feet from a pneumatic drill (which would be a relatively quiet 85 decibels), and as loud as operating a riveting machine, and it's almost as loud as the noise of a jet taking off 200 feet from where you're standing (120 decibels). A decibel level of 118 is enough to cause discomfort, while most people experience pain in the 140-decibel range.

"I've seen many young people, under 20 years old even, who are apparently suffering from severe hearing damage," says Cubbage. "People should be aware that sound over certain volume levels is going to cause hearing difficulties."

Musician Mark Coffey agrees. "I already have a little loss in my right ear from playing drums and cymbals as a kid," he says. "Now I wear cotton in my ears and I tape up my cymbals. But I wish someone would invent a cymbal that wasn't so loud."

Loudness, however, is part of what a lot of today's music is all about.

"When you're playing on stage with 400-watt stacks of Marshall amplifiers something happens," Coffey says. "It rattles your head and gets into your blood. And kids are coming for that charge, that volume, which has little to do with music. It's too bad, because they might be getting zapped by 130 decibels."

Alcohol Makes Things Worse

Mark Coffey has also observed that his hearing seems to deteriorate if he's been drinking.

"Loud restaurants really bother me now because I've noticed that if I've had a couple of drinks my hearing gets much worse. It's a lot harder to hear conversations in a noisy background if I've had something to drink."

Martin Robinette, Ph.D., professor of audiology at the University of Utah, and Robert Brey, Ph.D., professor of audiology at Brigham Young University, describe the connection between alcohol and hearing and explain why drinking increases an individual's risk of hearing loss.

"If you're in a disco, for example, and drinking, sound appears softer because of the deadening effect of alcohol," they say. "Consequently you want the sound to appear louder."

Tranquilizers or any other suppressant drug will cause the same reaction, according to Dr. Robinette. Furthermore, these substances make the auditory mechanism, which is designed to protect your ear, less effective.

"There are muscles in the middle ear that contract the eardrum when subjected to more than 90 decibels," Dr. Robinette explains. "With alcohol or common tranquilizers it takes more noise before the muscle contracts. And when it does finally react it's sluggish, not as effective in its contraction."

The young jogger we mentioned earlier hasn't been drinking and isn't on his way to a rock concert. His only source of potential hearing trouble lies in the earphones he's just put on.

According to the American Academy of Otolaryngology-Head and Neck Surgery in Washington, D.C., many portable headphone/cassette radios produce sound at levels greater than 100 decibels. Reversible damage to the inner ear can occur from listening at levels near the maximum output, and repeated exposure, the Academy points out, may result in permanent nerve deafness.

One in ten Americans suffers from some hearing loss, much of it caused by presbycusis, or hearing loss associated with aging. Injury and various diseases also contribute their share to deafness. But what is of particular concern to health-care professionals and to people in high-noise-level occupations is the ever-increasing number of Americans who are losing their hearing simply because of the noise they subject themselves to. It is estimated, for example, that 10 million Americans today suffer from industry-related, noise-induced hearing loss.

"Unlike many parts of the body that tend to regenerate, you really don't get back your hearing once it has been damaged," cautions Cubbage. "Therefore, people, regardless of profession, should take every step to protect their ears."

Protective Measures

Fortunately, there are certain precautions one can follow to help prevent hearing loss. For Cubbage, who spends most of his time in recording studios, the answer is simple: "I just don't turn the volume up full blast, especially when I'm using earphones. And when I'm someplace where prolonged exposure to loud noise might cause hearing damage—the target range, for example—I wear earplugs."

Earplugs are highly recommended by Dr. Abramson. Cautioning people to use silicone putty or foam plugs designed to protect against noise, not water, he says, "Good earplugs will attenuate the sound about 20 decibels. When you're subjecting yourself to any continuous loud sound like chain saws or power mowers, or even riding a noisy subway, you ought to protect your ears to avoid damage. Plugs are good. Earmuffs—the kind used by airport mechanics—are even better for prolonged exposure to loud noise such as using a chain saw."

Dr. Abramson also advises people to be alert to unexpected sources of high-volume sound. Some of the new cordless phones, for example, ring through the receiver, which could send 120 decibels straight into your ear if it happens to ring after you've picked it up. This is enough to cause permanent damage to susceptible people.

More and more people in noisy occupations are now making it a habit to protect their ears at work. For example, most of the workers at Argos Incorporated, a foundry in Brewster, New York, wear earplugs. A few prefer earmuffs, which they can pull on and off easily when they need to talk to somebody.

While rock 'n' roll audiences are not apt to start showing up at concerts wearing industrial earmuffs, there are some precautions they can take to protect their ears.

Dr. Abramson suggests concertgoers avoid standing directly in front of speakers. He further advises, "If you're at a concert or anyplace else where the sound is so loud you can't talk or if it's causing pain, you must leave that spot."

Signs of Damage

How to tell if a certain noise has damaged your ears? One warning sign is that any ringing or a muffled sound that lasts more than a few minutes indicates injury. If either of these conditions persists for more than a few days a hearing test is recommended.

"In today's technological society there is noise every-where," Cubbage reminds us. "In my own experience I've seen a lot of hearing damage caused by environmental factors, and I think this is much more serious than deterioration brought on by age. It's a shame, too, since much of it can be avoided."

What You Must Know about Triglycerides

If you're concerned about beating our nation's number-one killer, heart disease—and who isn't these days?—you probably have a sample of your blood analyzed periodically for its fat or lipid content. Such testing is an excellent way of predicting your risks for heart disease. And it lets you see for yourself, via computer-tallied numbers, just how well weight loss, healthy foods and exercise work to reduce the fatty particles found in blood that can clog arteries and cause heart attacks and strokes.

Cholesterol always seems to get top billing when it comes to listing the fatty substances in blood that cause heart disease. And cholesterol has earned its bad name. But along with it on the computer printout of your blood analysis you'll see another reading, this one for triglycerides.

We don't usually hear as much about triglycerides, per-haps because researchers are less certain about their role in heart disease.

One early analysis of data from the Framingham study, a long-term health survey of a Massachusetts town, found that, by themselves, triglycerides didn't seem to cause heart disease. But recently, with newer means of analysis, these same re-searchers have come to the opposite conclusion.

"New data shows that triglycerides *are* an independent risk factor for heart disease," says William Castelli, M.D., director of the Framingham Heart Study. "Anyone who has high blood lipids—cholesterol *or* triglycerides—should be con-sidered a high-risk coronary patient."

Older women should be especially concerned about high triglyceride levels, according to these new findings. "Our recent data showed that high triglycerides is a terrible risk factor in women," Dr. Castelli says. "As a matter of fact, in women over age 50, it's a better predictor of coronary disease than LDL cholesterol. Believe it or not."

Doctors do use triglyceride levels as an indicator of health status. They agree that low levels are a sign of good health because they almost always occur along with low levels of other harmful fatty particles, like cholesterol. They also agree that high levels are at least indirectly associated with an increased risk of heart disease, because they are invariably accompanied by high levels of other harmful blood fats. In other words, triglycerides may do their harm independently, at least in some people. But they almost certainly cause trouble in league with other forms of fat in the blood.

Fat Energy, Fat Storage

Triglycerides are the biggest of the blood's oily particles. They are composed of three long strings of fatty acids attached to a sugar-alcohol molecule. Triglycerides make up almost all of the group of blood fats known as very-low-density lipoproteins (VLDLs), which is a large fraction of the low-density lipoproteins (LDLs), the blood fats known to cause the most harm to the circulatory system.

Triglycerides do two things. They provide the body's major source of energy from fat. Most of the fat and oil we eat is composed of triglyceride molecules. And they are the body's main storage form of energy. Much of the fat, sugar or carbohydrates we eat that we don't quickly burn as energy is transported to the liver, converted to triglycerides and moved back through the bloodstream to be stored in voluptuous thighs or rounded bellies.

Our bodies' fat stores are not static, although they might sometimes seem as fixed as the Rock of Gibraltar. The fat moves in and out of the bloodstream as stockpiled supplies are burned up and new stores move in. The more fat we have encasing our bodies, the more we also have circulating in our bloodstream. That's why Don Mannerberg, M.D., of the Nutritional Preventive Medicine Clinic, Richardson, Texas, (and former director of the Pritikin Longevity Center in California) calls high blood triglycerides "a kind of internal fatness."

"Just as we can get fat under the layers of our skin and in our bodies, we can have fat blood, so to speak," Dr. Mannerberg explains in his book, *Aerobic Nutrition* (Hawthorn/Button, 1981.) That's also why most doctors agree the best treatment for high triglycerides is losing weight, along with exercise and dietary changes.

The Greasy-Spoon Effect

Triglyceride levels in the blood vary greatly from hour to hour, depending on food intake. After a large greasy or sugary meal, levels can rise dramatically and stay high for hours. That's why a triglycerides blood test is always done after an overnight fast.

Normal triglyceride levels are based on age and sex.

Today, most doctors agree that a "normal" range is from 85 up to 250 (milligrams per deciliter of blood). Mildly to moderately elevated levels, 250 to 500, pose double the risk of heart disease in people with other risk factors. And severely high levels, 500 and above, are usually a genetic problem, and can also increase the risk of heart disease if other risk factors are present.

Just how healthy "normal" triglyceride levels are is a matter of some debate. Because triglyceride levels do rise so much after a fatty meal, some doctors prefer to see lower fasting blood levels than those accepted by the American Heart Association (AHA).

"Studies have shown that triglyceride levels rise by as much as 120 points after a typical American meal of 40 percent fat and stay elevated for as long as nine hours," Dr. Mannerberg says. For people within the American Heart Association's normal range, this could mean triglyceride levels rising as high as 300.

That has Dr. Mannerberg concerned, because studies have shown that as triglyceride levels rise above 200, red blood cells begin to clump together. This clumping blocks capillaries, decreasing oxygen delivery to the tissues, particularly to the brain. In its most severe form, it can contribute to strokes and heart attacks.

"Studies by Meyer Friedman, M.D. [who first defined the 'type-A' personality], show that the ideal fasting blood level for triglycerides is 125 or less," Dr. Mannerberg says. "At that level, even if triglycerides rise after a fatty meal, they're not going to go high enough to cause clumping."

Some other doctors, though, including those on the National Institutes of Health (NIH) triglycerides panel, think there is an important difference between the "newly issued" triglyceride-rich particles that flood the blood after a high-calorie meal and "circulating" VLDL, which is present all the time, even during fasting.

They think the newly issued particles are less likely to cause coronary blockage because the molecules are whole, intact and unlikely to contain much cholesterol. The older circulating VLDL could be more harmful because it tends to contain bits of molecules that may more readily stick to artery walls. It also carries more cholesterol.

The Sugar Question

Perhaps the area of most dispute involves the effect of sugar on triglycerides. Some researchers think sugar is a major culprit in raising triglyceride levels. Others, notably a panel of blood-fats experts convened last year by the NIH, chaired by researcher Scott Grundy, M.D., Ph.D., of the Health Science Center, in Dallas, do not consider refined sugar a significant problem except as it contributes to obesity.

"It is true that all sugars raise triglyceride levels somewhat, and that refined sugars raise them a little bit more than complex sugars, such as starches," Dr. Grundy says. "But there is still some controversy about that. We're not absolutely sure." He thinks obesity, a high-fat diet and lack of exercise contribute more to heart disease than too much sugar.

Some physicians, though, put greater emphasis on sugar.

"I think it's fairly well accepted that in certain groups of people, even in amounts consumed in the typical American diet, sucrose or fructose-containing carbohydrates will raise triglyceride levels, sometimes significantly," says Sheldon Reiser, Ph.D., head of the U.S. Department of Agriculture's Carbohydrate Nutrition Laboratory, in Beltsville, Maryland.

Most likely to see this effect are people with non-insulin-dependent (type II) diabetes or a type of triglyceride-metabolizing problem. These people have high insulin levels when they eat sugar. They also have higher than normal levels of uric acid in their blood. For them, it's recommended to avoid refined sugars, Dr. Reiser says.

But other people might also want to think about keeping their sugar intake low, Dr. Reiser says. "Sugar and fat work together to raise the fatty components of blood more than would either alone. It's a synergistic effect. The dangers of sugar are increased if you add fats, and the dangers of fats are increased if you add sugars."

Some people, especially those sensitive to sugar, also have high triglyceride levels when they drink, and so should avoid alcohol, Dr. Mannerberg says.

Dr. Grundy agrees that alcohol can raise triglycerides, "but maybe not in the dangerous way that obesity and diabetes do. People with very high levels, 500 or more, are prone to pancreatitis, a painful, sometimes fatal inflammation of the pancreas that is aggravated by alcohol intake. They need to avoid drinking."

Most people whose triglyceride levels are above 500 have a genetic inability to properly metabolize this fat, Dr. Grundy says.

"There are actually two known conditions where very high triglycerides are found," Dr. Grundy says. In one type, the liver overproduces and pours triglycerides into the blood. This type apparently is associated with a high risk of heart attacks and pancreatitis.

In the other type, a normal amount of triglycerides is coming into the blood, but the body can't break it down normally, so blood levels remain high. "We don't think there is quite as much risk in this case," Dr. Grundy says.

But it takes complicated laboratory tests to determine which type you might have, and since in 80 percent of these cases it's a problem of overproduction, most doctors simply assume high triglycerides mean an increased risk for heart disease, Dr. Grundy says. Any evaluation should include an assessment of other risk factors, including other blood fat levels and a family history of early heart attack. Treatment for these super-high levels usually includes drugs to lower triglyceride levels and many of the diet and lifestyle changes mentioned below.

Treatment of Choice

What should you do if you're one of the millions of Americans whose triglycerides are moderately high, approaching 250 or more?

First, have three separate blood tests to confirm the diagnosis. "I do this to make sure the lab was correct and to establish a good baseline level before beginning treatment," Dr. Grundy says.

His treatment, in all but the most extremely elevated cases, begins with weight loss, exercise and dietary changes, not drugs. It's the same as both the NIH panel and the AHA recommendations, which Dr. Grundy helped establish. In most ways, it's the same sort of program you would follow to try to lower cholesterol levels and to reduce most heart-disease risks.

"I can't emphasize enough how important it is to lose weight," Dr. Grundy says. "Even ten pounds can help in people who are only 20 to 30 percent overweight. Any extra energy the body has that it doesn't need turns into triglycerides. The loose calories floating around in your body that you don't burn up are made into triglycerides."

And that's why exercise is so effective, too. One study found that ten middle-aged men with triglycerides of 180 or higher were able to lower those levels an average of 25 percent by jogging, doing calisthenics or playing handball for one hour three times a week for four months. And they saw this effect even though their body weight remained constant (*Atherosclerosis,* March, 1985).

There's no doubt that the typical high-saturated-fat, high-cholesterol American diet dramatically enhances triglycerides' potential for harm. "You should make fat 35 percent or less of your calories to reduce this effect," Dr. Mannerberg says. In overweight patients, there's no need to replace this fat with other calories. For people within a desirable weight range, the AHA used to recommend replacement with polyunsaturated fats. Now, however, it recommends complex carbohydrates.

Dr. Mannerberg includes additional treatment for some patients who don't respond well to weight loss, exercise and a lower-fat diet. They cut out all alcohol and sugar and change their meal patterns so they don't gorge at night.

"I don't do everything with everybody," he says. "A lot depends on the triglyceride level, other medical problems and what the patient can tolerate. I prefer to put the main emphasis on lifestyle and diet, then, if we need to, adding these other things as helpers."

He may have them eat fatty fish like salmon, or take fish-oil capsules. "There's good evidence that these oils lower triglyceride levels," he says. A recent study by doctors at the Oregon Health Sciences University found that triglyceride levels fell from 91 to 52 in people on diets rich in fish oils. Those researchers concluded that the effect was due to the fish oil's ability to inhibit the synthesis of a protein used in the production of blood fats, called apoprotein B (*Arteriosclerosis,* May/June, 1984). The NIH panel on triglycerides suggests fish oils deserve a closer look.

"I think of lifestyle changes as the first, and most important, means of treatment of high triglycerides in most people," Dr. Grundy says. "And it's important to give these things time to work. I'd give them several months to a year before considering drugs."

Understanding Dizziness and Vertigo

The world is whirling about your head and you feel like you're about to fall. It's a dizzying illusion, a masterful bit of sleight-of-hand perpetrated by your mind, your ears, your eyes and the muscles of your body, all conspiring to bring you to your knees.

Dizziness, even a wobbly moment or two, can be frightening. Alfred Hitchcock really knew what he was doing when he turned the world's movie-goers onto their heads in *Vertigo*.

We're all a bit dizzy from time to time. Some of us more dizzy than others. And while dizziness usually doesn't signal the presence of some underlying life-threatening illness, that unsteady state often is disabling, throwing not just your body but your whole life off balance.

Dizziness is an enigmatic symptom. Its causes are numerous and frequently pose diagnostic puzzles for doctors. On the plus side, most dizziness is treatable. If doctors can't completely stop the dizziness, often they can do much to alleviate other symptoms, such as nausea.

To understand dizziness, we first have to examine that marvel of human engineering, balance.

"The balance system is centered within the brain, and three major sensory inputs feed into that balance center," says Cecil W. Hart, M.D., associate professor of clinical otolaryngology-head and neck surgery at Northwestern University Medical School, in Chicago. "One is the labyrinth, which is rather like a gyroscope in the inner ear. Another is vision, where you see what's upright and what's horizontal. The third is proprioception, which is the sensation from your muscles, joints, the soles of your feet on the ground and things like that."

Anything that interferes with the orderly functioning of any one of these systems can upset the anatomical applecart, causing you to lose your balance. Conditions affecting the ears, the heart and blood vessels, the central nervous system or the body chemistry can disrupt the balance system. So can emotional disturbances.

"We had a dizziness clinic here at Northwestern for a couple of years," says Dr. Hart, who ran the clinic with David A. Drachman, M.D., a neurologist, now with the University of Massachusetts. "We found that there are about 63 significant diseases that cause dizziness. One-third of the patients' dizziness was based on diseases of the ear. Very few of these are life threatening. One-third seemed to be psychiatric, and these are not necessarily life threatening. And the other third were basically metabolic things, such as diabetes, multiple sclerosis and neurological diseases."

In fact, says Dr. Hart, many patients did not know they had multiple sclerosis or diabetes until their dizzy spells led them to seek medical help. "Dizziness often is the first symptom," he says. "We pick up many patients who come in here, and they've never seen a doctor or they've only seen their family doctor. You find that this is the first evidence that they've had of multiple sclerosis."

The doctor's first job is to find out what you really mean, by taking your vague complaint of dizziness and further refining it.

Sorting Out the Symptoms

"Dizziness can mean many different things to many different people," says Michael H. Stevens, M.D., associate professor of otolaryngology at the University of Utah School of Medicine, Salt Lake City. "If somebody says, 'I'm dizzy,' I'll ask him to use another word and redefine it for me so I can tell what he's experiencing. One of the difficulties we have in dealing with people with balance disorders is that they often have a hard time describing what they're experiencing. It's not that they're inarticulate, it's just that sometimes it's a difficult thing."

One very common balance problem often confused with dizziness is the specific symptom vertigo, described as a spinning or tilting sensation. Being merely light-headed or feeling weak and giddy, with a sensation of movement, may not be the same thing.

It isn't necessarily that vertigo is more serious than dizziness, but that the symptoms may point to completely different disorders. Vertigo is present in numerous inner-ear disorders. Certain drugs—diuretics, some antibiotics and caffeine—also may trigger a bout of vertigo.

Most vertigo stems from the ear, but not all. Severe head injuries, epilepsy, strokes and brain tumors also can cause vertigo.

Of all the disorders that cause vertigo, three—Ménière's disease, benign positional vertigo and vestibular neuronitis—are most common, says J. Cameron Kirchner, M.D., assistant professor of surgery in the otolaryngology section at Yale University Medical School.

Each disrupts your sense of balance. Here's how:

Ménière's disease affects all age-groups, says Dr. Cameron, but it's most common among middle-aged women.

It's unknown exactly what causes Ménière's disease, which produces changes in one ear, and sometimes both, touching off vertigo and often causing hearing loss. Ménière's sufferers also complain of tinnitus, or ringing in the ears, and a feeling of "fullness" in the affected ear. In time, after numerous attacks, serious hearing loss may result. This disease affects one in 1,000 people.

"The attacks can go on, each attack lasting a few hours at a time, for many years," says Dr. Kirchner. "They can be of sufficient frequency, up to two or three times a week, that the person can be severely incapacitated for long periods of time."

Treatment for Ménière's disease varies widely, according to Dr. Kirchner, including low-salt diets and the use of diuretics or vasodilators. Symptomatic treatment includes drugs to combat nausea, including anti-motion-sickness medicines.

If all other treatment fails, there are operations that can reduce or eliminate vertigo. One, for patients who still have good hearing, has a success rate between 50 and 80 percent. Another, for patients whose hearing is gone or nearly absent, is more successful—over 90 percent. But doctors might have to sacrifice whatever hearing is left in the affected ear to restore balance.

Benign positional vertigo is another inner-ear disorder where changes in head position cause vertigo. "People will notice, for instance, that they're okay during the day if they're up and walking around," says Dr. Kirchner, "unless they turn their head too rapidly to one side or until they lie down to go to bed at night. Then vertigo occurs.

"The vertigo in this disorder is characteristically very short, less than a minute, but it can be quite severe for that time, so severe that the patient is very frightened by it."

Benign positional vertigo is not to be confused with a common form of dizziness known as *postural hypotension*. In benign positional vertigo, the episodes of "spinning" last from 15 to 30 seconds and are caused by moving the head in a particular way. Postural hypotension, on the other hand, consists of a fleeting moment or two of unsteadiness after you've rapidly moved from one body position to another—for example, from lying down to sitting up.

Benign positional vertigo is triggered when microscopic calcium-carbonate stones inside the inner ear—used to detect linear movement—become dislodged, through aging or trauma. Viral infections can have a similar effect on balance. Postural hypotension is prompted by a transient episode of low blood pressure. More on this, later. Interestingly, an attack of benign positional vertigo can be repeated by simply repeating the movement that caused the first attack. However, says Dr. Kirchner, if the patient repeats the maneuver three or four times, the vertigo will lessen in intensity. But that doesn't stop the attacks altogether.

"If the patient doesn't put himself in the provocative position for the next half hour or so, then the next time it happens, he becomes very dizzy again.

"It is a benign disorder. In most cases, it's limited to a few weeks' duration before it gradually subsides, except in some elderly people, when it can be chronic."

Vestibular neuronitis is an inflammation of the vestibular nerve, usually triggered by a viral infection. "The attack is really one *long* attack of vertigo," says Dr. Kirchner. "It starts one day, gradually builds up and may take several weeks to subside. A person with vestibular neuronitis can be severely incapacitated, if it's a severe case, for that period of time."

Vestibular neuronitis is self-limiting: It goes away on its own, after lasting two or three weeks.

Two other causes of vertigo:

Labyrinthitis, an inner-ear infection, which may result in vertigo and hearing loss, and;

Acoustic neuroma, usually a benign tumor impinging on a nerve of the inner ear, causing tinnitus, hearing loss and, occasionally, vertigo. An operation to remove the tumor is recommended as a remedy.

Dizziness, like true vertigo, takes many forms. In the absence of the merry-go-round symptoms of vertigo, doctors must investigate other possibilities.

Dizziness can be the early warning sign of distinctly different health problems, some of them potentially serious, including *heart attack, cardiac arrhythmias, hypertension* and *atherosclerosis.* However, dizziness can also be brought about by *hypoglycemia* (low blood sugar) or *hyperventilation* (the rapid breathing that sometimes accompanies an anxiety attack).

Another cause of dizziness is the aforementioned *postural hypotension.* According to Dr. Stevens, this form of dizziness, which the patient might mistakenly describe as vertigo, is very common. Usually, it isn't a serious condition. Doctors advise patients to rise more slowly. However, if it is particularly severe or persistent, it is advisable for the patient to see a doctor.

"Dizziness of the non-vertigo variety—unsteadiness or light-headedness—probably is much more common than true vertigo," adds Dr. Kirchner. "Most people, at some time in their lives, feel light-headed for a moment or two. There are life-threatening problems that can cause dizziness, but those are very much the exception."

An Aging Problem

Although we all feel dizzy or light-headed from time to time, the elderly, as a group, are particularly prone to balance disturbances.

"The elderly do experience a number of balance problems, which are almost certainly related to the degenerative process," Dr. Kirchner says. Since dizziness and vertigo are caused by so many things, how is the average person supposed to know the difference between the serious and not-so-serious? Simply put, you can't. But in most cases, using tests designed to narrow down the possibilities, a medical specialist can tell you what's wrong.

Many otolaryngologists, or ear, nose and throat specialists, begin by culling clues from patient questionnaires. For example, Northwestern University's Dr. Hart utilizes a 30-page computerized questionnaire.

"In the questionnaire, we explain what *we* mean be dizziness and the various types of dizziness that can be included in that general, overall umbrella," says Dr. Hart. "You need to define the field a little bit for the patient before you discuss things with him, to make sure you're both talking about the same thing and you're on the same wavelength."

If the doctor still isn't sure what's wrong with you, he or she may ask you to undergo a hearing test and/or a more complicated test called an electronystagmogram, or ENG.

What is the ENG and how does it work?

"There's a very close relationship between the balance system within the inner ear and the movement of the eyes," says Dr. Hart. "You very often see abnormal spontaneous eye movements in patients who have diseases of the inner ear."

The ENG uses an electrical field to monitor eye movement. "What you do is hook up the patient and monitor the eye movements," says Dr. Hart. "As the eyeball moves, the electrical field moves. You look for spontaneous movements within the eye.

"The ENG can tell you whether there's a balance dysfunction to begin with. Secondly, it tells you whether it's within the ear or the brain. Thirdly, it may tell whether the disturbance is on the left side or the right side. And with some of the new techniques, you can localize it within various parts of the brain."

The eyes are monitored continuously while the doctor puts your balance system through its paces, rapidly moving your head from a prone to a sitting position, tilting your head from the left to the right and directing warm or cool water or air into your ear. These all are done to elicit a predictable response, to cause the eyes to move in a particular way. If your eyes don't do what they're supposed to do under those conditions—if they move in an unusual manner, move more than they should or not move at all—the medical specialist may be able to determine the nature of the disorder. But even ENG is fallible.

"If a person's test results are normal, that is of some diagnostic benefit," says Dr. Kirchner. "It doesn't necessarily mean that the person doesn't have a balance problem, because the ENG is an imprecise test. We don't have a good test or series of tests that can give us precise data regarding the balance system. This is something we've had a terrible time coming to grips with. For example, the water test really only tests one of the five balance organs of the ear. What we end up trying to do is to extrapolate from the integrity of that one to being able to make inferences about the integrity of the other ones, and that's a very poor system."

Nevertheless, the ENG can be useful in eliminating some of the more fearsome possibilities.

How dizzy do you have to be before you seek medical help? First, advises, Dr. Hart, ask yourself these three questions:

1. Is the dizziness severe?

2. Is it persistent?

3. Are there other alarming symptoms, such as chest pain or rapid heartbeat?

If you answer to yes to any or all of these questions, the experts say, you may require a doctor's diagnosis. Pay attention, in particular to the last question. If you have these symptoms, you may require immediate medical assistance, since dizziness, along with chest pain and other symptoms such as profuse sweating, can signal the onset of heart attack.

For most of us, a bout of dizziness is not a life-threatening emergency. Overall, doctors advise, use your common sense in deciding when to seek help.

"Everybody can get a little dizzy," reminds Dr. Hart. "How much pain requires a trip to the doctor? If you get a tummyache and it goes away, do you go to see a doctor? How often do you get a headache and how often do you see a doctor about it? I'd lump dizziness in the same category, really. If you have a significant amount of dizziness, if you think it's important, you should consult a physician about it."

Mojave Mouth

"When my mouth gets dry, my speech starts to slur. So when I'm at the bridge table and I try to say, 'I bid two no trump,' and it sounds like 'I play trumpet,' the girls know to get me a glass of water." Helen Rohlwing loves to play bridge. But for the past year, she's been having a problem with lack of saliva. "I've been to doctors, and they don't know what to do about it. They say it's caused by getting older. My feeling is, if I have to live with it, I have to live with it," she says. She jokes about the problem, but she doesn't like it much. "Chew gum, drink water and go to the bathroom. It's a great program. You ought to try it sometime; you won't like it."

According to Philip C. Fox, D.D.S., a senior investigator at the National Institute of Dental Research's Dry Mouth Clinic, xerostomia, or lack of saliva, is not an inevitable part of aging as Helen Rohlwing thinks. In fact, it's not necessarily related to age at all, since cottonmouthed people come in all ages—and in greater numbers than you might think. Dr. Fox estimates that at least 4 million Americans suffer from xerostomia for some period of time. But what causes this common problem? There are many reasons—maybe one that applies to you.

Xerostomia is a common side effect of drugs, says Minnesota registered pharmacist and health consultant Dianne Eberlein. (Dr. Fox estimates that this group may be around 3 million strong.) "Mood-altering drugs often cause dry mouth," says Eberlein. "These include antidepressant and antipsychotic drugs, as well as drugs for anxiety. Also, drugs used for Parkinson's disease, some drugs used for stomach problems and even common, over-the-counter antihistamines can cause dry mouth." She says the drug side effects may explain why many people think dry mouth is an inevitable part of aging—more old people than young people experience it, possibly because of the large amount of drugs older people often take. But young people sometimes take those drugs, too.

A possibly even more common reason for temporary dry mouth is garden-variety anxiety. "It's just one of those things that happens when you get anxious," says Robert Oresick, Ph.D., assistant professor of psychology and counseling at Boston University. "When you're nervous, the 'fight or flight' reaction is triggered. So your body's attention goes away from digesting food—the primary function of saliva—and goes toward dealing with the danger your body perceives," he explains.

Another common cause of dry mouth is as simple as bad breathing habits. Robert Spalten, D.D.S., director of Omnicare in New York City, says that people who habitually breathe through their mouths will experience chronic dryness. And many people experience a change in the composition of their saliva (this might occur for a variety of reasons) and, as a result, *feel* as though their mouths are dry. (The same *feeling* of dryness in a wet mouth can also be due to a neurological problem, says Dr. Fox.)

One of the more prevalent causes of dry mouth isn't too well known but, according to Dr. Fox, is experienced by at least 1 million Americans—it's an autoimmune disease called Sjögren's syndrome. (Autoimmune diseases are those in which the immune system works too hard and causes the body to react against itself, breaking down the tissues as though they were foreign bodies. This is just the opposite of AIDS, in which the immune system doesn't work *enough*.) According to Dr. Fox, Sjögren's syndrome affects the salivary glands, the lacrimal glands (which provide moisture to the eyes) and may also involve a connective-tissue disease such as rheumatoid arthritis, which is an autoimmune inflammatory disease. (Osteoarthritis is not an autoimmune disease and is not related to Sjögren's syndrome.)

Another all-too-common cause of dry mouth is radiation therapy involving the head and neck. "This will generally severely and permanently compromise the salivary function," says Dr. Fox. Also, says Ms. Eberlein, diabetics may have problems with dry mouth.

What Can You Do?

Even a small deficit of saliva can promote gum and tooth decay. But for most people, the main motivation for seeking help is that being a Sahara-mouth just isn't comfortable. Dr. Fox points out that what can be done depends upon the cause and severity of the situation.

"If there is absolutely *no* salivary function, as in some cases of Sjögren's syndrome," says Dr. Fox, "the glands cannot be stimulated. All you can do is treat the symptoms." There are so-called saliva substitutes that can be bought over the counter in drugstores, but Dr. Fox does not feel they are more effective than frequent sips of water or other sugarless drinks, especially when eating. "It's important that it be sugarless because of the major problems with tooth decay in these people."

Dr. Fox also points out that the somewhat common use of

saline solution to give relief from dry mouth is probably a mistake. "Drinking a saline solution won't hurt but won't do any more good than drinking water," he says. "But rinsing the mouth with it could actually be drying and would just make the situation worse."

Most people have some salivary function and can do more. If dry mouth is due to nervousness, relaxation is your best bet. "If you're someone who experiences a lot of anxiety, you might want to examine why," says Dr. Oresick. "For relief of dry mouth, though, you could relax yourself by thinking of peaceful scenes or consciously tensing and relaxing your muscles. Tranquilizers just augment the problem," he adds.

If the dry mouth is drug related, you might want to consult your physician about switching medicines. Discontinuation should allow the salivary function to return, though Dr. Fox warns that prolonged use of the drug could permanently reduce or stop the saliva flow in your mouth.

Mouth breathers should see an ear, nose and throat specialist to determine why they are breathing through their mouths. If your mouth is often open even when you have nothing to say, you could have polyps in your nasal passages. Or maybe you just never learned to breathe through your nose. But it's not too late to acquire the skill. And you'll probably be glad if you do, because, as Dr. Spalten says, "The more you breathe through your mouth, the dryer it will be."

Possible New Treatment

If you and your physician aren't sure why your mouth is dry, but you know you want it wet again, there are ways to stimulate salivary flow.

Dr. Fox, at the Dry Mouth Clinic, is currently experimenting with pilocarpine, a drug that is normally used in prescription eyedrops to lower the pressure of the eyes. In the mouth, it has an entirely different effect. So far, the clinic has used the drug to increase people's saliva flow for up to three hours, and is now shooting for eight. Dr. Fox says, however, that the drug won't be on the market for another year or two.

Until then, there are non-drug-related ways to stimulate flow that will work for just about everyone.

Dr. Spalten recommends biofeedback to teach self-control of the salivary flow. He also suggests increasing the flavoring of your food, sucking on sugarless lemon or lime candy, or even putting clean pebbles in your mouth. Dr. Fox has found that both the taste and chewing action required by sugarless gum help salivary action. And some people respond well to carbonated, sugarless fluids. He also recommends lemon or lime flavors because they chemically induce saliva, but warns that the high acidity of these fruits can etch the teeth and irritate the mouth, so they shouldn't be overused.

Sugarless mints are a good alternative, he says. And, of course, drinking six to eight glasses of water a day can only help.

Preventing Cervical Cancer

It's probably happened to someone you know, or perhaps it's even happened to you. Instead of the postcard or phone call from your gynecologist's secretary, you get an ominous call from the doctor himself. "Your Pap smear wasn't quite normal. I'd like to see you again in my office." Despite his reassurances, your mind spins with questions and dark imaginings. This is a time when you need all the information you can lay your hands on.

The Pap smear takes a scraping of cells from the cervix, the tip of the uterus that extends into the vagina. The sample includes cells from the cervix, vagina and uterine lining (called the endometrium). The cells are checked by a laboratory for any signs of abnormal change and classified according to the degree of abnormality found.

The Pap smear can usually detect inflammation or infection of the cervix and endometrium, which can occur with intrauterine devices, pelvic-inflammatory disease or *chlamydia* infections. It is not as useful for detecting cancer of the endometrium or ovaries.

But it is of great value in detecting possibly precancerous changes on the cervix long before any signs are visible to the doctor's eye. These changes are known as cervical dysplasia. (Dysplasia simply means "abnormal development of cells.")

Currently, Pap smears are categorized one of two ways: either (1) placed into five classes and several subclasses according to the severity of tissue change, or (2) increasingly, the abnormality found in the cells is more fully described.

Class I is a normal smear with no abnormal cells. Class II is a kind of catchall category of minor cell changes that can include inflammation and infection or very early signs of dysplasia. Class III includes mild and moderate dysplasia. These are also known as cervical intraepithelial neoplasms (CIN) 1 and 2. (Neoplasm means "new and abnormal tissue growth, which may or may not be cancerous." Intraepithelial means "among the cells" lining the cervix.)

Class IV Pap smears include severe dysplasia and cancer confined to the lining of the cervix, both called CIN 3. Class V is invasive cancer—cancer that has spread beyond the cervix to the uterus and possibly other parts of the body.

Always Ask Why

While it's important to know into what class or category your Pap smear has been placed, it's even more crucial to know *why* it's been put there, says Ralph Richart, M.D., director of the division of obstetrics and gynecologic pathology and cytology at Columbia-Presbyterian Medical Center in New York City.

"The current classification system is simply not precise enough to keep up with new knowledge of the cause and process of cervical dysplasia," Dr. Richart says. "Every doctor should request from the laboratory a written description of the cell changes found in the Pap smear. And he should be able to explain in detail to his patient the reason for the abnormality, especially in the catchall Class II category."

The cervix may be reacting to a vaginal infection like *trichomonas,* or to uterine inflammation from an IUD. More important, it may be showing signs of exposure to one of the viruses that cause venereal warts that have been associated with cancer. Since treatment varies in each of these cases, these distinctions are crucial. Unfortunately, they are not always made, Dr. Richart says.

A Sexually Transmitted Disease

The whole school of thought concerning cervical dysplasia and cancer has been turned upside down in the last year or two as the result of findings that many of these tissue changes are caused by a group of sexually transmitted viruses known as Human Papilloma Virus (HPV), or, commonly, as the condyloma virus, Dr. Richart says. If they are allowed to flourish, all these viruses will cause abnormal tissue growth or breakdown. Some will form tiny flat warts that can grow undetected on the cervix, in the vagina or male urinary opening or on the penis. Others form large cauliflower-shaped warts.

"It is now generally agreed that the condyloma virus is the major agent responsible for abnormal Pap smears," Dr. Richart says. "The genetic material of this virus has been found in a large percentage of dysplastic tissue samples."

The condyloma viruses are named by numbers according to their order of discovery. There are approximately 40 now known. "Several of them—particularly HPV 6 and 11—are thought to be essentially benign," Dr. Richart says. "Their association with neoplasia is not very strong."

On the other hand, HPV viruses 16, 18 and 33 are routinely associated with cancer and cancer precursors. The main sign of exposure to these viruses is the development of flat genital warts, which often go undetected until they're discovered during a gynecological examination in women, or a penile exam in men.

Practically all abnormal Pap smears show signs of the condyloma virus. One percent of all women, 2.5 percent of women under 30, and about 4.5 percent of women in high-risk groups have the virus detected by the Pap smear.

"Recent studies have not confirmed the original suggestion that herpes is a factor in cervical dysplasia or cancer, and I believe most authorities now believe that herpes plays no or only a minor role," Dr. Richart says.

What's a high-risk group? "The most important risk factor

is multiple sex partners," Dr. Richart says. "It's just like any other sexually transmitted disease. Every time a woman climbs into bed with a new partner or a man climbs into bed with a new partner, they run the risk of that person being a carrier of this virus. Every other risk factor is secondary."

The statistics confirm that sexual activity plays a major role. Among nuns, cervical cancer is rare. Among prostitutes, it's almost an occupational hazard. And there's an unfortunate increased risk for the one-man woman whose mate tends to roam, as seen in Latin America. In those countries, tradition dictates that wives be strictly monogamous. But there's an equally strong tradition for men to frequent prostitutes. In those countries, cervical cancer rates are high.

And there's an especially disturbing risk factor for some other women. The wife of a man whose previous wife died of cervical cancer is herself three times more likely than normal to develop the disease.

Obviously, these findings point to the need for the woman who is diagnosed as having dysplasia to insist that her husband or boyfriend see a doctor, too. In fact, one study, by researchers at Columbia University, found that 53 percent of the male partners of women with cervical dysplasia had condyloma lesions on their penis or in their urinary opening. This could be especially important in cases where the virus returns again and again.

"A woman who has recurrent infections probably should have her husband checked to see if he is a carrier, but that's ahead of where we are now," says Rosemary Zuna, M.D., director of cytopathology in the department of pathology at the State University of New York, Stony Brook. "It's probably the thing to do, but it's not being done routinely at this time."

While researchers believe the condyloma virus triggers most dysplastic symptoms, they also think other risk factors may make some people more vulnerable to the virus, or may trigger forms of dysplasia that are not virus-related. "We know that in some women, these lesions go away by themselves," says Dr. Zuna. "And we know that in some women they develop into cancer. What we don't know is the real key that causes some lesions to actually invade the tissues and become malignant."

Tobacco is a known risk factor. Women who smoke more than 15 cigarettes a day are twice as likely as nonsmokers to have cervical dysplasia or cervical cancer. And they are 3.5 times more likely to develop invasive cancer (*British Journal of Cancer,* January, 1985). Samples of cervical mucus taken from women smokers contain chemicals that cause cancerous cell changes (*American Journal of Epidemiology,* September, 1985).

The daughters of women who took the drug diethylstilbestrol (DES) during pregnancy may be a high-risk group. But women using birth control pills or menopausal estrogen are apparently not at risk.

It's true that there have been one or two English studies linking the use of birth control pills with cervical dysplasia. But many top researchers contest their findings. "These studies are criticized because they did not adequately take into account the increased sexual activity that might be seen in women using birth control pills," Dr. Richart says. "When this factor is controlled for, these women seem to develop no more cervical dysplasia than normal."

Women who choose diaphragm and condom use may have lower than usual cervical-cancer rates, possibly because the devices protect the cervix from contact. Male circumcision is no longer considered a factor. Nor is the number of children you have had, or a family history of cervical cancer.

Poor Nutrition as a Risk Factor

Until recently, eating habits were not considered an important factor in cervical dysplasia. Now, though, researchers are finding that nutritional status apparently plays a role in the development of cervical dysplasia and cervical cancer, just as it may with other cancers or precancerous conditions. Poor nutrition may make cervical cells less able to withstand the mutagenic effects of some viruses or the carcinogens found in the cervical mucus of women who smoke. It can also weaken the body's immune system, making it less able to fight infection.

Lower-than-normal intake of selenium and vitamins C, A,

and the B-complex vitamin folate have been found in women with cervical dysplasia or newly diagnosed cancer.

Researchers at the Albert Einstein College of Medicine in New York City found that women whose intake of vitamin C was less than 30 milligrams daily (only half the Recommended Dietary Allowance, and equal to about half a medium orange or two ounces of juice from concentrate) had a risk of developing cervical dysplasia ten times greater than that of women whose daily intake was higher (*American Journal of Epidemiology*, November, 1981).

They also found that women were three times more likely to have severe cervical dysplasia or cervical cancer if their vitamin A intake was below the group median of 3,450 international units daily (equivalent to about a third of a cup of shredded carrots or four dried apricots).

"Whether nutritional factors and their interaction in cervical epithelial cells have antitumor properties that may influence the host's immune system or even influence the maturation or development of normal cervical epithelium is a challenging scientific problem," says Seymour Romney, M.D., director of gynecologic cancer research at the Albert Einstein College of Medicine.

Dr. Romney is currently involved in two research projects. In one, women with mild or moderate dysplasia are being given supplemental vitamin C to see if their condition improves. In another, they are being treated with topical applications to the cervix of a synthetic form of vitamin A, retinyl acetate gel. "We have no results yet on these studies," Dr. Romney says. But researchers at the University of Arizona may have an inkling of what to expect. They did a study very similar to Dr. Romney's vitamin A study, using a different form of vitamin A, transretinoic acid. The treatment showed encouraging activity in preventing worsening of the condition in women with mild to severe cervical dysplasia.

Folate also seems to play a role in dysplasia, especially in women using birth control pills, who may have lower body levels of this vitamin, according to researchers at the University of Alabama at Birmingham.

Their research involved 47 young women with cervical

dysplasia. Half were given 10 milligrams of folate (25 times the RDA) each day, while the other half received a placebo (dummy pill). After three months, the cervical dysplasia had regressed to normal in four of the women in the folate group. There was no improvement in the placebo group. In fact, the dysplasia had worsened in four of the women. (Note: Large doses of vitamins require a doctor's supervision.)

"Just what kind of nutritional recommendations will come out of further research is yet to be seen," Dr. Romney says. But the indications are now that preventing cervical dysplasia is yet another good reason to make sure you're getting plenty of vitamin C and A-rich fresh fruits and vegetables, and folate-rich dark leafy greens.

It may be frightening to find yourself in the high-risk group. But there are two important—and reassuring—things to remember about Pap smears. First, quite a few women at some time in their lives will have smears showing mild, moderate and even severe dysplasia. And they won't go on to develop cancer. Their condition will be successfully treated.

Second, if you're getting Pap smears every year, it's very unlikely that you'll suddenly discover you have cervical cancer. Most cell changes in the cervix follow a long, slow continuum. Most cervical cancers take about ten years to develop, and appear years earlier as treatable dysplasia. The women who end up with invasive cancer either do not get yearly Pap smears or are among the unlucky few who develop a rapidly growing cancer.

How your doctor treats your cervical dysplasia depends on several factors—the classification of your smear, whether you intend to have children, other risk factors, your doctor's own opinions and experience, even how reliable you are at coming in for follow-ups. Nevertheless, there are some generally accepted procedures for diagnosis and treatment, Dr. Zuna says.

If your smear is Class II, your doctor should determine the reason for the classification and treat it. Inflammation or infection can be treated with antibiotics or other drugs.

However, if your smear shows signs of the condyloma virus, treatment is needed, whether the dysplasia is mild, moderate or severe. "Some doctors will wait a few months and do another smear, but I'd rather get a firm diagnosis and treat," Dr. Richart says. "It's a sexually transmitted disease, whether you currently have symptoms or not. Why risk infecting someone else?"

Treatment is basically the same for all classifications of dysplasia.

First, your doctor will view the cervix with a colposcope. This instrument provides a magnified view of the cervix, allowing the doctor to see growths, from which he will take a small bit of tissue for biopsy. "A biopsy is important because it's the only way to rule out invasive cancer," Dr. Richart says.

If no growth is seen, but another Pap smear still shows abnormal cells, you doctor will probably want to do a conization, Dr. Richart says. "Conization is usually done when you cannot absolutely rule out the possibility of invasive cancer." In the procedure, a cone-shaped piece of tissue is cut from the center of the cervix for analysis. This may reveal a lesion in the cervical canal. The procedure usually does not affect your ability to bear children.

If either of these procedures confirms dysplasia or exposure to the condyloma virus, the treatment is the same—the lesions are removed. They are treated just as are some forms of skin cancer. They can be coated with chemicals that make them slough off, frozen in a procedure called cryosurgery, vaporized with a laser beam, or, less frequently, burned off with cauterization.

Several months later, you have a follow-up Pap smear. If it is not normal, the treatment may be repeated. If it is normal, you and your doctor will determine a schedule of smears to monitor for possible recurrences. Even though your condition is cured, you are now in the high-risk group and should have Pap smears at least once a year.

How Often for Pap Smears?

The American Cancer Society now recommends that most women have a Pap smear only once every three years, after two initial normal smears. The American College of Obstetrics and Gynecology still recommends a smear every year.

There are two good reasons for an annual Pap smear. One is the remote possibility that you may develop a fast-growing cancer. The other is that the Pap smear does have a 15 to 30 percent rate of error of false negatives—that is, it indicates your cervix is normal when it isn't. More frequent tests minimize your chances of walking around with an undetected dysplasia.

Dysplasia occurs most often in women aged 25 to 35; cancer in situ (confined to the uterus) in women 30 to 40; and invasive cancer, in women aged 40 to 60. Women who have had a hysterectomy should still be getting regular Pap smears, Dr. Zuna says. The cells in the upper vagina can develop cancer, and sometimes partial hysterectomy is done, leaving the cervix. A Pap smear doesn't always detect cancer of the endometrium or ovaries. Always inform your doctor of any abnormal bleeding or pain, even if your Pap smear is normal, Dr. Zuna says.

Medical Care Newsfront

New Weapons against Cataract

When she reached the age of 79, Agnes Andrews, a spry, high-spirited woman who lives in Richfield, Connecticut, decided that she'd suffered with her cataracts long enough. "I had to have people help me down the stairs, not because I was weak but because I couldn't see the steps," she told us recently. "I couldn't see colors either. I told my daughter I'd bought a new black coat, and she said, 'Mother, that coat is purple.' I couldn't stay at a book long either, and I love to read."

But making the decision to have cataract surgery wasn't easy, she admits. "I think everybody is scared at first," she says. "I know the fear that people have about anything touching their eyes. And many older people say that since they're so close to the end, they might as well live with it."

Mrs. Andrews found the courage not to live with it however. In May, 1984, she had one cataract removed. The other came out a year later. Both operations were successful, but in one of her eyes the tissue behind her lens implant fogged over, clouding her vision a bit. That made her a candidate for the new Yttrium-Aluminum-Garnet (YAG) laser, which her doctor used to cut a hole in the tissue.

"I had a funny feeling about the laser. But it surprised me," she says. "It was just as though I was having an eye exam.

It looked like snow for a moment. It was short. There was no pain and no after-effects—except good ones."

Like thousands of other elderly and not-so-elderly Americans, Mrs. Andrews benefited from the new surgical techniques now in use among the nation's ophthalmologists. To be sure, not everyone's treatment is as successful as hers. But these new therapies have helped thousands avoid the sense of helplessness and despair that poor vision or blindness bring.

The argon laser, the YAG laser and phaco-emulsification— these are the newest procedures. They are mustered against the four most common sight-destroying diseases among people over the age of 45. These are: macular degeneration, glaucoma, diabetic retinopathy and cataract.

The new therapies have streamlined much eye surgery to the point where it can be performed on an outpatient basis. And though none of them constitutes a cure, they can often prevent or arrest the effects of eye disease, and have offered help where once there was none at all.

The Blue-Green Laser

If you suffer from diabetic retinopathy or macular degeneration, an ophthalmologist may already have introduced you to the argon, or thermal, laser.

Both of these ailments cause, for complex reasons, the weedlike growth of abnormal, unnecessary blood vessels on or below the surface of the retina—the inside lining of the eye that receives images and sends them to the brain. When these blood vessels multiply or, worse, if they rupture and leak, they can cause blindness.

That is where the laser comes in. It "spot welds" the abnormal vessels before they can do much harm. When the ophthalmologist (who sits opposite you in a darkened room and looks into your eyes with specialized contact lenses and a modified microscope) fires either a few or several hundred split-second bursts of blue-green light into your eyes, each burst creates a tiny burn. The burn dries up the unwanted blood vessel.

This sounds dangerous, but ophthalmologists say it isn't. The laser will neither destroy your eye, we're told, nor burn a hole through the back of your head. To understand why not, think of the way you burned holes in dry leaves with a pocket magnifying glass when you were a kid. The laser works much the same way. It heats only the spot it's focused on, and only for a split second. Think of it as a very sharp cauterizing iron made of intense aquamarine light.

Unfortunately, the argon laser can't help everyone. Some eye patients are better candidates than others. Lee M. Jampol, M.D., chairman of the ophthalmology department at Northwestern University School of Medicine, told us that diabetics who seek early treatment have the best chance, but only 10 to 20 percent of those with macular degeneration can be helped.

"It's important for all diabetics to have regular eye exams," he says. "If we catch the retinopathy in the early stages, we have a good chance of success. The problem is that if you wait until there are symptoms, such as a detached retina or bleeding in the eye, it might be too late." If caught early, the laser can reduce the risk of blindness in diabetics by as much as 70 percent.

In macular degeneration, there is only a small "window of opportunity" for treatment after the first symptoms appear. "In this disease a person will develop blurry vision and distortions," Dr. Jampol says. "Straight lines will appear curved. He will lose his ability to read. If we catch it right away, the laser can seal off the abnormal blood vessels. But success is variable. Some people are permanently cured. Some have recurrent symptoms within a year or two."

But, in at least one study, the argon laser cut the amount of vision loss in one group of macular-degeneration patients by half (*Western Journal of Medicine,* February, 1984).

The laser does present a few hazards. John H. Mensher, M.D., of the Mason Clinic, Section of Ophthalmology, in Seattle, told us that after extensive laser treatment to the retina, some diabetic patients lose some of their night vision. At times the laser may hit a sensitive spot and cause a stab of sharp, brief, dentallike pain. (If a large amount of laser treatment is performed, a local nerve block is given so that the treatment is pain-free.) In rarer cases, the laser light may damage the macula—the center of the retina—and cause permanent partial vision loss. Also, the various types of laser treatments may temporarily raise the pressure in the eye to glaucomalike levels. Therefore, your doctor may have to check the intraocular pressure after treatment.

Some people find argon laser treatment uncomfortable, others don't. It's been compared to having a green flashbulb go off in your face a hundred times. Many people have a headache and light sensitivity afterwards, and have to lie down when they get home, depending on the reason for, type and amount of treatment. If you go for laser therapy, have someone drive you home.

The Argon Laser and Glaucoma

Four to 5 million Americans suffer from glaucoma, a potentially blinding disease in which pressure builds up inside the eye and pinches the optic nerve. The pressure comes from a backup in the flow of fluid. Watery fluid normally enters and exits the eye at all times, but it gets backed up when something clogs up the "drain," called the trabecular meshwork. With too much inflow and too little outflow, pressure mounts.

Three out of four glaucoma patients can control this pressure with special eyedrops. For the rest, an ophthalmologist might suggest 80 to 100 bursts of argon laser. No one knows why, but the laser sometimes opens up the trabecular meshwork and unclogs the drain.

Harry Quigley, M.D., chief of the glaucoma service at Johns Hopkins University School of Medicine, in Baltimore, told us that some people are better candidates for this kind of therapy than others. "Your chances are best if you are elderly, if you have never had eye surgery before, and if you have what is called primary, open-angle glaucoma," says Dr. Quigley. "In two-thirds to three-fourths of these patients, pressure will go down."

There is a rarer form of glaucoma, called angle-closure glaucoma, for which the laser has also been used. While open-angle glaucoma progresses without symptoms, angle-closure glaucoma causes blurry vision, red eyes and pain. To treat it, ophthalmologists use the laser to puncture the iris—the colored part of the eye—so that fluid flows freely between two chambers in the front of the eye and pressure drops. "If you catch this early enough, the laser will cure it," Dr. Quigley says.

Ophthalmologists are now using three new and different surgical techniques to restore vision in cataract patients. The procedures are extracapsular cataract extraction, phacoemulsification, and the YAG laser treatment.

In extracapsular cataract extraction—the most popular form of cataract removal—a surgeon makes a small, curved incision in the eye, reaches, inside and removes the front part of the lens, the anterior capsule. This exposes the hard inner part of the cataract, the clouded nucleus.

The nucleus is removed by gentle pressure, causing it to slip out like a watermelon seed squeezed between the thumb and forefinger. A suction device then removes the rest of the cataract, intentionally leaving the back capsule, or lens-encasing membrane, intact. (This part is used to support the new artificial implanted lens.)

Phacoemulsification is a somewhat controversial and relatively new cataract operation that removes the clouded nucleus a different way. The surgeon makes an even smaller incision in the eye, then inserts a hollow titanium needle into the lens. The needle vibrates 40,000 times a second, simultaneously liquefying the cataract and sucking it out.

Phacoemulsification is attractive because it requires a smaller incision and fewer stitches than extracapsular extraction. But the operation requires specialized training and very expensive equipment and is more difficult to perform.

For that reason, make sure the surgeon is well trained in this method of cataract removal.

"Don't be someone's first or second patient with phacoemulsification," says Julius Shulman, M.D., a New York ophthalmologist and author of *Cataracts, The Complete Guide from Diagnosis to Recovery, for Patients and Families* (Simon and Schuster, 1984). "It's more difficult operation with more complications. Call the chief eye surgeon at your hospital and find out who is experienced. Phacoemulsification should be your doctor's primary technique."

The "Buck Rogers" Laser

The YAG laser can be an important addition to extracapsular surgery. In 20 to 30 percent of cataract operations, the back capsule (which was left in to support the new artificial lens) becomes clouded again and obscures good vision. Before the YAG laser, surgeons were often forced to leave in the fogged-up, vision-reducing capsule or risk a second operation to open it. Now, however, they can use the YAG laser to cut a hole through the capsule in a microsecond.

This "scalpel of light" fires vaporizing bursts that last a billionth of a second or less, earning it the nickname of the "Buck Rogers" laser.

"The YAG causes a mini-explosion at its point of focus," says ophthalmologist Jerome Levy, M.D., of the Manhattan Eye, Ear and Throat Hospital, in New York. "Using it is like being able to put a knife in your eye without putting a knife in your eye."

The result is dramatic—a person can walk in severely visually handicapped and leave a few minutes later with near-perfect vision, all because the YAG blasted through the clouded capsule.

The YAG can be used in other kinds of eye surgery, replacing both knife and operating room. It's the most exciting laser now in use. "People say it's a miracle, and I admit, it is a bit of a miracle," says Dr. Levy, whose nurses, no matter how many times they've seen it, still like to go down the hall and watch a patient's transformation.

There are one or two experimental developments in ophthalmology that may make eye surgery easier in the future. One is the silicon lens. Now under review by the U.S. Food and Drug Administration, this lens flexes in the middle, making it possible to slip it into the tiny incision the surgeon makes while performing phacoemulsification. One reason phacoemulsification is impractical now is that the surgeon has to widen his incision anyway for the eye to receive today's inflexible Plexiglas lens implants.

Ophthalmologists have also been talking about something called the excimer laser. According to one doctor, the excimer can cut very precisely and may become the first laser to be used to do radial keratotomy, an eye operation to correct myopia.

"Safer Than Ever"

Is eye surgery right for you or for someone you know? Ophthalmologists say that it has never been safer to perform eye surgery than it is today. Many patients say it isn't as painful or complicated as they thought. Just ask someone like Mrs. Andrews.

"It has enhanced my whole life," she said of her cataract operations. "I feel young again. I travel all over now. In fact, I'm flying down to St. Thomas to visit my daughter. I know the fear that people have about their eyes. But if you know anyone who has cataracts have them call me. I'd say, 'Go for it!' "

Breathe Deep, Breathe Easy

When's the last time you had to stop to catch your breath? Were you climbing a mountain? Blowing up balloons for a birthday party? Looking at price stickers on this year's new cars?

Most of us don't think much about it until we come up short—when we have to drop whatever it is we're doing and struggle to suck in all the air we need. Then, we might wonder: Is this normal? Is it happening because I'm getting older, or am I out of shape? Or, if you consider yourself physically fit, you might ask: Am I pushing myself too hard?

It's well that you should wonder, and perhaps see a doctor who can help determine the cause of your shortness of breath and what you can do about it. Being able to breathe easily doesn't just mean your lungs are fit. It's also an important indicator of your general good health and your level of fitness.

Just how accurate an indicator your lungs are of your health status was studied recently by doctors analyzing data from the Framingham study, a 27-year-long medical study of a Massachusetts community. The researchers looked at the results of a simple, inexpensive procedure, called a spirometry test, given to each person in the study. The test measures the amount of air expelled from the lungs in one quick deep breath. This is known as "forced vital capacity," and it can be an important figure because it's the standard measure by which doctors gauge the health of your lungs.

Spirometry is most often used to confirm a diagnosis of lung disease, such as emphysema or chronic bronchitis. Doctors at the Mayo Clinic in Rochester, Minnesota, say it beats a physical exam or x-rays at detecting lung disease, and that smokers aged 35 and older should have this test every five years to determine if there is lung damage. And the Framingham researchers discovered that the test shows even more.

"We found that the lung's forced vital capacity is indirectly related to the rate of all cardiovascular diseases and to overall mortality," says William B. Kannel, M.D., a Boston University professor of medicine and a heart specialist. "The lower someone's forced vital capacity, the more likely he was to go on to develop heart disease or to die early. In fact, it turns out to be one of the strongest predictors of life expectancy, even competing with major cardiovascular risk factors like smoking or high blood pressure."

Dr. Kannel also found that a below-normal score on the forced vital capacity test was an especially good early predictor of heart failure in people who showed none of the typical symptoms, like fatigue, swollen ankles . . . and shortness of breath. The test picked up this sign of impending failure even before patient or doctor was aware of it.

"Most doctors regard this lung test as a useful index of the severity and progression of heart failure once it has begun," Dr. Kannel says. "But they don't realize they could also use it to detect patients with vulnerability to heart disease. That's unfortunate, because too often by the time symptoms become apparent, the heart is too worn out to be saved."

It is true that many people who do poorly on the forced vital capacity test don't have heart disease. They have chronic lung disease caused by smoking, says Robert Hyatt, M.D., director of the Mayo Clinic's Pulmonary Function Laboratory. And the test is underutilized to detect even this, he says. "It could detect lung disease in smokers early enough to do something about it, but most doctors don't use it for that. I'd say the average patient has lost half of his lung function by the time he sees a doctor for shortness of breath."

But nonsmokers who do poorly on the test or whose test results are unclear for lung disease could get further screening with a heart function test called an echocardiogram, Dr. Kannel says. This painless ultrasound scan can determine the amount of blood that flows through the heart with each beat. It can tell you if your poor lung function is due to a weak heart.

What does the heart have to do with the lungs? If the heart isn't pumping as efficiently as it should, blood begins to back up in the lung's millions of tiny capillaries, making them stiff and swollen with retained fluid, and reducing their ability to expand and contract. A failing heart also hinders the lungs' ability to oxygenate blood, as fluid buildup around the lungs' tiny cells prevents the close contact between blood and air needed for oxygen to move into the blood. The result is a painful gasping for air that can't be used anyway.

Exercise and Oxygen Use

People can perform normally on the forced vital capacity test, have no signs of lung or heart disease, but still find themselves short winded. Their problem is too much knitting and not enough cha-cha-cha. They're out of shape.

"And their lungs really have very little to do with their being short of breath," says Bryant Stamford, Ph.D., director of the exercise physiology laboratory at the University of Louisville's School of Medicine. "One of the big misunderstandings about exercise is that when people become winded they are having problems with their lungs. That's just not the case. Healthy lungs have a tremendous excess capacity. They have no problem moving enormous amounts or air or diffusing all the oxygen they can hold into the bloodstream. They can keep up with any physical activity. It's almost impossible to overload them."

Then why the huff-and-puff schtick? Because there are other links in the oxygen-bearing chain that can slow us down, Dr. Stamford says.

Take the bloodstream, for example. "Can the blood carry enough oxygen? Here you are dependent on the number of red blood cells and the amount of oxygen-carrying hemoglobin they contain," he explains. In this case, the most common problem would be anemia, most likely caused by an iron deficiency. Iron is an essential part of hemoglobin. Without it, oxygen can't move through the bloodstream, tissues are deprived and so a feeling of breathlessness occurs, often accompanied by rapid heartbeat. Getting the iron you need is important to your exercise program, because exercise helps to promote a slight increase in blood volume and number of red blood cells. Provided enough iron is available, this makes your blood better at carrying oxygen.

And can the heart pump enough blood? "The heart is probably the primary bottleneck in the oxygen-delivery system," Dr. Stamford says. "If you are not aerobically trained, the best way for the heart to circulate blood is to beat very often. That's just not very effective, and it stresses the heart."

An aerobically trained heart, on the other hand, begins to pump more blood with each beat, during exercise and at rest. It becomes a more muscular, efficient pump, and is less stressed. It allows you to be more active without running out of breath.

The muscle tissues are the final link in the oxygen chain. Muscle tissues that aren't getting enough oxygen send a message to the lungs—breathe more! But that doesn't help. The lungs are already providing plenty of oxygen.

What does help is exercise, Dr. Stamford says. Exercise promotes the development of good capillary channels to the muscle tissues, making sure the blood gets where it's needed. It increases the number and size of tiny energy-producing mitochondria in the muscle cells, making them more effective oxygen users. And it increases the amount of a substance found in the muscles, myoglobin, that escorts oxygen from the bloodstream into the cells.

Endurance Building Takes Time

So how do you take advantage of all these stamina-building goodies? It takes some time, and possibly some perseverance,

Dr. Stamford admits. It means you have to exercise strenuously enough to deliberately make yourself short of breath, to create an oxygen demand all the way down to your muscles.

"You need to do aerobic exercise at least 30 minutes at a time, three or four days a week," Dr. Stamford says. The first few weeks you'll certainly feel your body screaming for the oxygen it can't get, but after several weeks, the links in the chain begin to tighten up, and you'll find yourself gaining stamina, perhaps even enjoying the exercise.

If you're over 30, are overweight, or become breathless even while inactive, you should see a doctor before beginning an exercise program, Dr. Stamford says. You want to make sure you don't have a heart condition that could be aggravated by exercise.

Can You VO₂?

Although people who are aerobically trained tend to have above-normal vital capacity, the FVC test won't measure your degree of fitness or ability to use oxygen. For that, you need a VO_2 Max test. The VO_2 Max test measures your body's oxygen consumption during exercise. It's not often done, though, except for research purposes or to satisfy the curiosity of superathletes.

And you don't really need to have it done, doctors say. It might be better, and it's certainly less expensive, to learn to monitor your body's oxygen needs yourself, pushing just a little further each time you exercise. But be careful not to overdo it. You be the judge and back off if you are breathing too hard.

"If a doctor is reasonably sure his patient is simply out of shape, he might put the patient on an exercise program and see if his stamina improves," Dr. Hyatt says. "If it doesn't, it becomes more of a diagnostic problem, and the doctor might then go to formal exercise testing, including the VO_2 Max test."

It's true that your lungs' vital capacity and your body's ability to use oxygen decrease as you age. On average, your vital capacity drops about 5 percent with each decade of life, mostly due to loss of lung elasticity. But it drops much faster in people who smoke, and may drop slower in people who get regular aerobic exercise, contends Dr. Kannel.

Maximum oxygen uptake also stays higher in people who exercise.

"In most people who find themselves becoming breathless, it's because of a lack of fitness, not necessarily aging," Dr. Stamford contends. "In our society, it's not difficult to find 30-year-olds who are huffing and puffing."

If fact, a 50-year-old endurance runner can have the stamina of a sit-at-home 18-year-old, although that's not to say the same runner does as well at age 50 as he did at 18.

"We do know there's something more than exercise involved, although we don't really know what it is," Dr. Stamford says. "Even though our marathoner continues to train, he will see a progressive decline in capacity over the years."

But chances are he won't see a debilitating decline. You don't have to run marathons to stay fit enough to function, Dr. Stamford says. "Even gentle exercise will help older people regain stamina. I think sometimes the best thing to do is walk, and just try to go a little bit farther each day."

Don't wait until you're blue in the face to think about where your next breath is coming from. Like most health problems, here again, prevention pays off.

Better Ways to Deal with Gallstones

Gallstone surgery is the most commonly performed operation in the United States. That should come as no surprise to anyone who has experienced the excruciating pain of a typical gallbladder attack. Who wouldn't willingly, even gratefully, march off to surgery for relief, especially with the knowledge that one agonizing attack may lead to another?

Gallstones afflict over 20 million people in the United States—about 4 percent of the adult population. They are the reason for 500,000 operations each year. Three percent of men and 10 percent of women between the ages of 50 and 62 will have a significant problem with stone disease.

Most gallstones are about the size of a marble, but they

can vary from a fine, gravellike substance to a one-inch-diameter boulder. And while many never cause any trouble, others can trigger intense pain, fever, infection, jaundice, peritonitis and pancreatitis—life-threatening conditions.

What determines who will get gallstones? "There seems to be a familial tendency to form gallstones," says Michael S. Gold, M.D., chairman of the department of gastroenterology at Washington Hospital Center and associate professor of medicine at George Washington University School of Medicine, in Washington, D.C. "Certain ethnic groups have a fairly high incidence—Pima Indians and Latin Americans. In other populations, there are general rules about who gets gallstones. They seem to occur more in women, in middle-aged people, in obese people and in women who've had many children. In medical school we used to call it the four F's: fat, fertile, female and forty."

Casting Stones

Doctors don't know exactly why or how gallstones form, but they do know that they originate from bile, a thick yellow liquid that's needed for the digestion of fats. Bile is produced in the liver, then passes into the gallbladder, a teardrop-shaped sac, where it is concentrated and stored until it's needed. When we eat, a hormone stimulates the gallbladder to contract, squirting bile through ducts and into the duodenum, the uppermost part of the small intestine.

"Bile is made up of a number of dissolved substances that have the potential of precipitating out to form stones," explains Dr. Gold, who also serves as vice president for medical education at the American Digestive Diseases Society. "The three important solids in bile are cholesterol, lecithin and bile salts, which are a derivative of cholesterol and are made in the liver. Those substances exist in little packages called micelles. It's a way of dissolving cholesterol in a water milieu (cholesterol is not readily soluble in water). The lecithin forms layers or plates, and the cholesterol droplets are in between the layers, like a marble sandwich. The bile salts encircle the package like a cellophane bag.

"These substances coexist in a very delicate balance.

When the relationship is disturbed, the cholesterol begins to slip out into crystals, and the crystals begin to accumulate in layers—like rolling a snowball."

How do the constituents of bile get out of balance? "If the liver makes less bile salts or more cholesterol, that might cause a stone to form," says Dr. Gold. "Obese people may get more gallstones because their cholesterol metabolism may differ. People with diseases of the small intestine, such as Crohn's disease, or those who've had a portion of the small bowel called the ileum removed also have a higher incidence of gallstones. That's probably because those areas of the bowel are where bile salts are absorbed to be reused later."

Women who've had many children may get gallstones for another reason. "During pregnancy, a hormone is secreted that causes the gallbladder to contract less than normal," Dr. Gold told us. "When the bile is standing still—a condition called stasis—there's a greater chance for cholesterol to crystallize and build up stones. Estrogen use may cause gallstones for the same reason. The point is that there may be several different mechanisms."

Squeeze Play

Trouble starts when, following a meal, the gallbladder contracts down, pushing a stone into the neck of the gallbladder and blocking the opening pipeline called the cystic duct. That squeezing down behind the obstruction is the pain of gallbladder disease. "The attack may be transient," Dr. Gold told us. "If the stone falls back into the gallbladder, the pain will subside and everything will be fine."

If the stone remains there, however, the obstructed gallbladder will begin to produce more and more fluid inside until it becomes a big distended bag. Then there are several possibilities. If the pressure inside is too great, the blood supply may be cut off. Then gallbladder will rupture. If the blood supply is only partially compromised in the wall of the gallbladder, the stone may fall away and the attack may subside with some fever or infection. Then a scar will form, the gallbladder will become shrunken and won't function normally, and more stones may form.

But if the stone is small enough, it might be squeezed through the cystic duct into the bile duct, where it blocks the bile coming down from the liver. When that happens, it's usually quite painful; the person usually turns yellow with jaundice, and has infection and fever.

"Sometimes the attack is so bad that we have to get the person to surgery right away," Dr. Gold told us. But if it's a routine attack, it might be better to wait and do the surgery on an elective basis.

Not all gallstones cause problems, though. In fact, a majority of gallstones are actually painless. "There are a lot of people who never know they're walking around with gallstones in their gallbladder," says Dr. Gold.

So how do we know that silent stones actually exist? They're discovered during x-rays for some other problems, or they may be found at autopsy.

Until recently, doctors didn't really believe there was such a thing as silent gallstones. Many doctors felt that eventually all stones caused problems and patients with gallstones were referred for surgery to prevent the "inevitable" future complications.

But a recent study by William A. Gracie, M.D., and David F. Ransohoff, M.D., of the University of Michigan School of Medicine and Case Western Reserve University School of Medicine, is changing medical opinion. One crucial finding is that none of the people with untreated silent gallstones in their study died because of their gallstone disease. Few ever developed problems, so few needed surgery.

Those who did develop pain tended to have no complications, so they were able to have low-risk elective surgery. And when pain did occur, it tended to be soon after the discovery of the stones, permitting elective surgery at a time when the risk was still low. In addition, the doctors found that the yearly risk of developing pain decreased with the passage of time.

"We conclude that innocent gallstones are not a myth, and that in some populations the majority of silent gallstones are inconsequential," say the doctors. "We believe that routine prophylactic operation for silent gallstone disease, at least in white American men, is neither necessary nor advisable" (*New England Journal of Medicine,* September 23, 1982).

The Sword and the Stone

When *is* surgery indicated? "Opinion varies," says Dr. Gold. "It's very controversial. But there's probably the beginning of a shift in medical philosophy."

"Results of a study carried out in the 1940s showed that about 50 percent of people with cholesterol gallstones eventually developed symptoms," points out Thomas Q. Garvey III, M.D., a gastroenterologist from Rockville, Maryland. Eventually many of these people required surgical intervention. And since elective surgery is much safer than surgery during complications, it used to be if you found gallstones, you'd recommend surgery.

"More recent studies suggest that, in fact, silent gallstones may tend to remain 'silent'—that is, they don't usually cause symptoms. There are several natural histories of gallstones. One of these, and it's pretty common, is a single attack which results in a diagnosis and then nothing—never another attack. It appears that up to 80 percent of people in whom gallstones are found may never have symptoms."

There are, however, several sorts of gallstone patients for whom surgery is still recommended. "If a patient is diabetic, elderly, or regularly spends a great deal of time far from adequate medical facilities, there is a relatively strong rationale for prophylactic gallbladder surgery," Dr. Garvey told us. "There is also a rationale for removing a large solitary gallstone, because such stones tend to cause complications and because there is an association between them and the development of gallbladder cancer. Whether these large stones cause cancer is unclear, and the risk of cancer is not great, but it's probably enough to recommend surgery. Further, surgery seems appropriate if the patient has intractable pain or has had episodes of inflammation of the gallbladder, bile duct or pancreas.

"If the patient is not having symptoms, does not have a large solitary stone, is not diabetic, and has ready access to adequate medical care, it might be wisest to watch and wait."

At this point you might be wondering just how someone goes on living *without* a gallbladder. "Very easily," says Dr. Gold. "We really don't miss it at all. Bile is still made in the liver, and circulates through the bile duct into the intestine."

One interesting point about gallbladder surgery is that it's only 85 percent effective—15 percent of the patients who have surgery continue to have pain. "There are several reasons for that," Dr. Gold explains. "First, the pain may not have been due to gallstones in the first place, Maybe the doctor saw the gallstones and decided to take them out, but the pain may have been caused by something else. Second, in the past, doctors didn't always check the ducts when they removed someone's gallbladder, and so they may have left some stones behind. But that happens less than it did in the past, because they are routinely looked for today. The third possibility is that years later, the person may re-form a stone in the bile duct. It's rarer, but it does happen."

Scope It Out

A new technique can handle precisely that situation—without surgery. It's called endoscopic retrograde cholangiopancreatography, or ERCP. To locate the stone, the doctor passes an endoscope, a flexible tube, up to the opening of the bile duct. Then the doctor injects a radiopaque dye and observes the filling of the duct under a fluoroscope. Once the doctor has identified the stone, he or she can open up the muscle at the end of the bile duct and remove the stone.

"The procedure is called a sphincterotomy," explains Jerome H. Siegel, M.D., assistant clinical professor of medicine at Mount Sinai School of Medicine and chief of gastroenterology and endoscopy at St. Clare's Hospital in New York City. "We pass an electrified wire through the endoscope and use it like a knife to open up the sphincter muscle at the end of the bile duct. The we take out the knife and put in a special catheter to remove the stone. One type of catheter has a balloon at the end. We pass the catheter past the stone, then inflate the balloon and pull it back, gently pulling the stone into the duodenum, where it passes out of the body with the fecal contents.

"People can live with diseased gallbladders," says Dr.

Siegel, "but they can't live with an obstructed bile duct. Over half a million people have gallbladder surgery each year. Twenty percent of those people require exploration of the bile duct to take out stones. If we see them first, we can take out the stones in the bile duct and their doctor can deal with the gallbladder later. That's important because morbidity and mortality rise significantly the longer the surgery lasts—the longer they have to explore the bile duct—especially in people 65 and over. If the surgeon can go in and just remove the gallbladder, the patient's hospital time and complications will be reduced."

To perform the procedure, the patient's throat is sprayed with an anesthetic and he or she is given a twilight sleep—not general anesthesia. "They're really out of it though," says Dr. Siegel. "Most patients don't know that the procedure is taking place. The endoscope is passed through the mouth, esophagus and stomach, and into the duodenum. Then the catheter is passed into the opening of the bile duct, the cholangiogram [x-ray] is obtained and the stone is removed."

Etched in Stone

"The procedure is less dangerous than surgery because the belly isn't opened up and there is no general anesthesia," continues Dr. Siegel. "And the convalescence is much shorter— about three to four days in the hospital. And most patients can resume their normal activities when they leave the hospital— they don't have to wait for an incision to heal.

"We have estimated that the endoscopic procedure costs only about one-fifth as much as the surgical procedure, when you look at time in the hospital and time lost from work," Dr. Siegel points out. Surgery just to remove the gallbladder may entail a hospital stay of one week to ten days. If exploration of the bile duct is done at the same time, the hospital stay may be two to three weeks. "If the gallbladder has stones in it, theoretically it's diseased and most doctors feel that it's going to be a problem," he says. "But we've found that about 90 percent of the people we've treated with the gallbladder intact have not had to have their gallbladder removed."

One of the most important things about the endoscopic procedure is that it's a permanent fix. While stones can be retained after gallbladder surgery, or re-form in the bile duct, that doesn't usually happen after a sphincterotomy. That's because the opening of the bile duct is permanently enlarged. If the duct is open and the bile is flowing freely, there's not enough stasis for the development of stones. "It's the best preventive treatment available against developing further stones in the bile duct," Dr. Siegel says.

Dissolve Your Troubles?

A few years ago, a new drug for dissolving gallstones got a lot of press. "Chenodeoxycholic acid is a naturally occurring bile acid that dissolves cholesterol and bile," explains Dr. Garvey. "But unfortunately, when given in the relatively high doses required to dissolve cholesterol gallstones, the drug causes a high incidence of therapy-limiting diarrhea. 'Cheno' can also cause significant liver damage in a not-inconsequential proportion of the patients to whom it's given. Further, gall-stone dissolution with 'cheno' takes up to two years, and only a small proportion of patients (about 15 percent) will experience dissolution. Chenodeoxycholic acid is on the market now with extremely restrictive labeling and its use is thought appropriate only in patients who are poor candidates for anesthesia or surgery itself, such as an older person with cardiorespiratory disease.

"In general, if you are dealing with complicated stone disease and you think the patient can tolerate surgery and general anesthesia, you recommend surgery.

"A closely related drug, ursodeoxycholic acid, is much more promising," Dr. Garvey asserts. "It appears to cause no liver toxicity, and does not cause diarrhea. It is currently on the market in Europe, and a new drug application will soon be submitted to the Food and Drug Administration for approval to market ursodeoxycholic acid in the United States. However, 'urso', like 'cheno', dissolves stones slowly, and in considerably less than half the people to whom you give it."

For years the standard therapy for patients with gallstones was to eat a low-fat diet. A meal with high fat content, doctors reasoned, would make the gallbladder contract more strongly, increasing the chance of it forcing a stone into the ducts. But a study done at Georgetown University School of Medicine has raised doubts about that approach. The doctors compared how the gallbladder contracted and ejected bile after volunteers ate meals containing differing amounts of fat. The results? "We conclude that the gallbladder dynamics in response to various meals are independent of a meal's fat content" (*American Journal of Gastroenterology,* October, 1984). But many doctors have found low-fat diets effective in preventing attacks and still recommend them.

There is some evidence that diet may have a role in preventing gallstones in the first place, but as yet the information is sketchy. "It seems highly likely that gallstone formation is influenced by diet," says Dr. Garvey. "But just how important dietary factors are and in what ways they exert these influences, nobody knows. Data relevant to this come from Japan, where prior to World War II the prevalence of cholesterol gallstones was very low. Subsequently, however, it has begun to approach the prevalence in Western societies. The only thing anybody can think of to explain this is dietary changes."

A recent study done at the University of Oxford in England addressed that issue. The researchers compared the prevalence of gallstone formation in vegetarian women with the prevalence in women who eat meat. They found that the meat-eaters had about twice the incidence of gallstones. "Vegetarians tend to eat less saturated fat in addition to not eating meat and have a higher intake of fiber than nonvegetarians," the doctors note. "These data suggest that some dietary factor associated with vegetarianism affords a strong, independent protective effect against this common condition . . . " (*British Medical Journal,* July 6, 1985). Further research may bring those factors to light.

Diabetes Alert!

It's estimated that 5 million of the more than 12 million diabetics in the United States don't realize they have the disease. And often the ones who do learn the truth do so almost by accident: A routine medical exam detects the disorder that no one suspects.

"Most people with undiagnosed diabetes are type II, those not dependent on insulin," says Robert C. Cantu, M.D., chief of neurosurgical service at Emerson Hospital in Concord, Massachusetts, and author of *Diabetes and Exercise* (E. P. Dutton, Inc., 1982). "Their symptoms (which can include excessive thirst, frequent urination, infections that won't heal, blurred vision and fatigue) are often so mild that they may not pay much attention or simply not connect them with diabetes."

But the price of ignorance can be high. Over time, diabetes—even with fairly mild symptoms—can affect every system in your body, slowly setting the stage for classic complications: heart and blood-vessel disease, impotence, eye trouble, nerve damage, foot problems and kidney disease. Ignoring diabetes and thus failing to control it increases the risk of all these maladies. And turning your back on the disease can forfeit your chance to force it into remission.

The Sugar Blues

For nearly three centuries it's been known that diabetes has something to do with sugar in the urine, but this is only a small part of the story. Diabetes mellitus (the full name) is a disorder of too much sugar, or glucose, in the blood. Glucose, the body's primary fuel, is always circulating in the bloodstream, feeding the body's cells with the help of the hormone called insulin. But in diabetes, either there isn't enough insulin to go around or the cells have trouble making use of insulin. The result is that glucose can't get into the cells and thus starts piling up in the blood—often "spilling over" into the urine.

Especially in the kind of diabetes called type I, all this may provoke yet another metabolic mixup. "When insulin is deficient or the cells are not using it properly, not only does the blood sugar build up, but if this process is unchecked (as in uncontrolled diabetes), the body breaks down fat and protein in an attempt to provide energy," says Peter A. Lodewick, M.D., a New Jersey diabetes expert and author of *A Diabetic Doctor Looks at Diabetes* (RMI Corporation, 1984). "This breakdown of fat forms acidic toxins, resulting in the condition known as ketoacidosis, which can be life-threatening to a diabetic."

So ultimately it's the starvation of cells and the flash flood of blood sugar that seem to give rise to the typical symptoms and acute complications of diabetes. Sugar in the urine causes frequent urination, which in turn leads to dehydration and extreme thirst. Weakness, hunger, weight loss, nausea, blurred vision—these too may arrive in the wake of the metabolic crisis. And if it rages out of control long enough, serious diabetic complications may appear.

This crisis, however, can vary in how it starts and the way it's controlled, depending on the type of diabetes. Up to 90 percent of diabetics have type II diabetes (non-insulin-dependent) —which is the easiest kind to control and the most likely to be nudged into remission. In type II, the problem is not so much that insulin is absent, but that its levels are low or it's not being used efficiently to ease glucose into the cells.

This form of diabetes used to be called adult-onset diabetes because it usually shows up in people over age 40, but it can also afflict younger people. At the time they're diagnosed, 60 to 90 percent of type II diabetics are overweight or have a history of being overweight, which suggests an important clue to countering their disease.

"Many overweight type II diabetics can lose their diabetes by losing weight," says Stanley Mirsky, M.D., president of the New York affiliate of the American Diabetes Association and author of *Diabetes: Controlling It the Easy Way* (Random House, 1985). "Sometimes a loss of even a few pounds is sufficient to accomplish this miracle. Losing weight may enable your body to either produce enough of your own insulin to keep your blood sugar normal or increase the number of cell receptor sites so that the insulin you produce can be utilized properly."

The other major form of the disease (there are also several rare kinds) is type I, or insulin-dependent diabetes, accounting for about 10 to 20 percent of all known diabetes cases. As the name implies, type I diabetics produce so little insulin that they need regular insulin injections. Unlike type II diabetics, people with type I are usually lean or have recently lost weight, are prone to ketoacidosis and endure symptoms that have come on strong and fast. And though type I can strike at any age, even as old as 70, its prime targets are young people under age 20, which is why it used to be called juvenile-onset diabetes.

Nailing Down the Diagnosis

So do you really have diabetes? Only your doctor can tell you for sure—and only after running the right tests (more about these in a moment). Testing is the only way your doctor can make the diagnosis and distinguish between true diabetes and other glucose problems.

One such problem is the condition known as impaired glucose tolerance (IGT). Its aliases include borderline, chemical, latent and asymptomatic diabetes—all terms now considered outmoded because they imply that diabetes is present when it really isn't. IGT's only sign is a blood glucose level somewhere between normal and diabetic.

IGT, however, is not something you'd want to ignore. About 25 percent of people with the problem eventually get true diabetes, and they seem to be at greater risk for developing atherosclerosis. On the other hand, it's possible to head off IGT's plunge into diabetes through diet, weight loss and exercise.

In nondiabetics, hypoglycemia (low blood sugar) isn't nearly as serious. (It can, though, be a severe reaction in some diabetics.) "Hypoglycemia is not dangerous," says Dr. Mirsky, "but it can make your life miserable. The symptoms may (and may not) include general weakness, fatigue, inability to concentrate, listlessness, butterfly sensations in the stomach and subnormal temperature. Also, rapid heart rate, shakiness and palpitations, sweating and apprehension. As someone has described it, it's as if you have almost been hit by a train."

But, says Dr. Mirsky, most nondiabetic people who suspect that they're hypoglycemic probably aren't. "No diagnosis of hypoglycemia can be made," he says, "unless low blood sugar and specific symptoms *occur simultaneously.* "This happens most in diabetic people using insulin, but fails to occur in a lot of would-be hypoglycemics.

At any rate, if you have diabetic symptoms, or you're pregnant or obese, or there's someone in your family tree who's had diabetes, the American Diabetes Association says you should be tested for the disease.

The old standard urine test, however, can only hint at diabetes—it won't yield a definitive diagnosis. Nowadays, doctors can get to the bottom line with blood tests, usually done after you've gone for at least eight hours without food or after ingesting a measured amount of glucose.

"With these blood tests," says Harold Rifkin, M.D., president of the American Diabetes Association, "physicians can determine with a high degree of certainty whether a patient has diabetes mellitus."

The Power of Deterrence

These days doctors are also doling out a lot of good news about the fight against the disease. To the diabetic, they point out that diabetes may not be curable, but it is manageable. To the person who fears getting the disease, they assert that in most cases it's preventable. Also, 20 to 30 percent of diabetics never get serious complications.

"Through proper diet, exercise and sometimes medication or insulin, diabetes is controllable," says Philip Raskin, M.D., professor of medicine at University of Texas Health Science Center in Dallas.

And the chances of deterring the disease altogether are even better. Scientists don't know for sure what causes diabetes, but they do know that some people seem predisposed to developing it. A family history of diabetes and obesity are major predisposing factors. And at least in type II diabetes, the most prevalent kind, you can take steps to successfully counter these influences.

"If you're predisposed to type II diabetes," Dr. Mirsky told us, "you can greatly decrease your risk by keeping your weight down. This implies, of course, a calorie-controlled diet and a sensible program of exercise. Such an approach can actually stop diabetes before it gets started."

For More on Diabetes

You can contact an affiliate of the American Diabetes Association. There are affiliates in every state, all with local chapters that offer plenty of information and support for people with diabetes and their families.

For the address and phone number of your state affiliate, call the American Diabetes Association diabetes information service center toll-free, 800-ADA-DISC.

Bioelectrical Healing Report

In 1974, Edward Sloboda nearly lost his legs when he was pinned between the bumpers of two vehicles. Four years later, the upstate New York building contractor was still hobbling around on crutches. The bone in his left leg just wouldn't heal, and lingering infections made a successful bone graft unlikely.

That's when Sloboda decided to try electricity, then a still-experimental treatment, on his fracture. He'd heard about it from a friend's doctor. "I was willing to try anything," he says. At that point, his only alternative was grim—amputation.

Sloboda became a subject in an experiment being conducted by Andrew Bassett, M.D., director of the Columbia-Presbyterian Medical Center's Orthopedic Research Laboratory, in New York City. Dr. Bassett has been studying the biological properties of electricity for more than 25 years.

Dr. Bassett has developed a bone-healing device that produces a special kind of electrical current generated by a pulsating electromagnetic field. Two molded plastic cups encase the broken limb on either side of the fracture. Inside are coils of wire charged with a special form of alternating current. The current creates a field of pulsating energy that causes an electrical current in the bone. The current is so weak most patients feel nothing. Wires lead from the cups to equipment the size of a book. (Another electrical bone-healing device uses surgically implanted electrodes threaded through the cast.)

Healing with these devices isn't necessarily fast. Edward Sloboda spent a total of 2,100 hours on his machine—almost nine months of up to 16 hours a day. But x-rays showed his bone had begun to heal within six weeks. And that's a wink of the eye when you're dealing with fractures that are years old. "We've even healed 40-year-old unhealed fractures," Dr. Bassett says. Both his method and the surgically implanted wires have about an 80 percent success rate. They have had government approval since 1979.

How Does Electricity Work?

Researchers know the body normally has tiny electrical currents flowing throughout. These currents are created by the flow of electrically charged particles called ions. In the body, ions are usually of calcium, potassium, sodium or magnesium. They flow in and out of the body's cells.

These currents start at the moment of conception, and seem to guide development and differentiation in the cells of the growing fetus. They also perform some remarkable feats in lower animals. For instance, they seem to be involved in the process that allows a salamander to regrow a severed limb or an eel to heal its cut spinal cord. In all animals, including man, the electrical current changes measurably when an injury occurs.

Scientists like Dr. Bassett believe these currents act to control many chemical events in the body. Messages they send to cells influence their growth and function.

"It's a kind of cellular Morse code," he says. "If you say dot-dot-dot to a cell with an electrical pulse, it's going to do one thing. If you say dash-dash-dash, the cell's going to do something else."

Much of the research work in this field involves "decoding" naturally occurring electrical messages so researchers can either mimic the messages or thwart them with a countercurrent to generate a particular type of cellular response.

In a fracture that won't heal, for instance, the process of normal repair has stopped with only half the job done. New cartilage has united the bone ends, but it is soft and unable to bear weight. It hasn't been hardened with calcium.

"We send an electrical message to the bone cells—'Look, you forgot to calcify that bloody mess in there. Do it now,' " Dr. Bassett explains. "If you deliver the right message in there, the cells carry out that particular step, and once that has happened, you have taken away the impediment to the final sequences of fracture repair."

The method is not used for fresh fractures, Dr. Bassett says, not only because it's not needed, but because the correct messages needed to speed natural healing are only partially understood. It's used only on fractures that have not healed for at least four months.

Dr. Bassett has also developed a way to stop bones from crumbling after certain injuries or from metabolic disturbances. In a condition called osteonecrosis, the blood supply to the hip joint is cut off by disease or trauma. This causes part of the joint to rapidly lose bone and collapse, resulting in crippling arthritis. But a certain kind of electrical stimulation, produced by circular pads worn on the front and back of the pelvis, prevents the loss of bone and coaxes the growth of new blood vessels into the affected part of the joint.

Additionally, Dr. Bassett is helping to develop electrical devices that one day may be used to stop osteoporosis in older women, or to prevent "space bones"—the loss of bone that weightless astronauts experience.

Other Tissues, Too?

Bone is the only tissue scientists have proved can be healed with certain forms of electricity. Bone-mending machines are the only kind of medical electrical devices on the market allowed by the government to make "healing" claims. But preliminary research indicates that other tissues besides bone may respond to certain electrical currents.

Work by William D. Stanish, M.D., chief medical officer of the Canadian Olympic team and assistant professor of medicine at the University of Dalhousie, in Halifax, Nova Scotia, seems to show that the same sort of current used with electrodes implanted in bone can also improve the rate and quality of healing in torn ligaments and tendons.

In athletes who required knee surgery, Dr. Stanish implanted a tiny titanium battery. A wire going from the battery was wrapped around the repaired ligament or tendon. Six months later, the knee was checked and the battery removed. The tissue grew around the wire with no problems.

Compared to people with similar injuries without an implant, Dr. Stanish found that his patients with implants had increased stability in the knee joint, faster healing times and stronger tendons.

"It's very exciting," Dr. Stanish says. "The fact is that

tissues do seem to respond when you supply electricity to them." However, he warns that no currently marketed electrical devices have been proved to heal tissues. "If you're thinking about using one, be very much prepared to look at the science behind it, not just the commercial allegations," Dr. Stanish says.

In fact, research with cells in culture indicates that soft tissue like muscle and skin should respond to specific kinds of electrical currents, says Robert Becker, M.D. Author of *The Body Electric* (William Morrow, 1985), Dr. Becker is considered one of the pioneers in the modern medical use of electricity.

"The rate of cell division can be speeded up in any tissue by the use of certain electrical currents," Dr. Becker says. "It's important, though, that the cells be dividing—growing or attempting to heal. And the electrical frequency must be a pulsating electromagnetic field with a frequency faster than that which occurs naturally."

Short-Circuiting Pain

Certain electrical devices do have government approval for use as painkillers. One of the more commonly used is the transcutaneous electrical nerve stimulator (TENS) unit. With this device, electrodes are taped to the skin over major nerves leading from the painful area and connected to a small battery that can be worn on the belt.

TENS units are used for many kinds of discomfort, especially chronic lower back pain, nerve irritation in the stumps of amputated limbs and aching from cancers of the pelvis, head and neck, says Stephen Butler, M.D., of the University of Washington's Pain Center in Seattle. Sometimes, too, electrical stimulation is produced by implanting electrodes in the spinal cord or specific areas of the brain.

"The applied electrical current seems to block the natural electrical current flowing through the nerves that is carrying the message of 'pain' from the site of injury to the brain," Dr. Butler says. "Although it doesn't work for every victim of chronic pain, electrical stimulation works very well for some, and it's always worth a try, especially when you consider the possible side effects of strong painkilling drugs." (For more information on TENS units and their applications, contact the Pain Control Network at 800-833-9911.)

Nerves truly seem to be the body's major pathways for electrical currents. And nerves that are hurt seem to respond to stimulation from certain outside electrical currents.

"Some regeneration of peripheral nerves does occur naturally," Dr. Bassett says. "However, we have found that in using the right kind of electrical messages we can double the rate at which this occurs. We can cut in half the amount of time it takes to restore normal function in animals with severed peripheral nerves."

Normally, in no mammal can the spinal cord repair itself. But in some lower animals, the spinal cord can heal quickly with the aid of natural electrical currents, Dr. Bassett says. He hopes that understanding how this process works may one day help scientists to regenerate spinal cords in creatures that have lost that ability, perhaps even humans.

After any injury, for example, there is what researchers call a "current of injury." When the spinal cord of a lamprey eel is severed, this current is carried into the cut region by a flow of calcium and sodium ions. The injury current is so strong that it could probably light up a flashlight, observes Melvin Cohen, Ph.D., professor of biology at Yale University.

"Initially, this current is so large we think it is further injuring the cells," Dr. Cohen says. "For instance, it's known in spinal-cord injury clinics that during the first week after the initial injury, secondary deterioration spreads from the site and may actually cause more damage to the spinal cord than the initial injury."

Dr. Cohen and his coworkers have been able to reduce significantly the amount of secondary injury to the spinal cord in lamprey eels by applying an electrical current in opposition to the current of injury. "Much more work must be done before this kind of thing can be tried in humans," Dr. Cohen says. "But now, we can create a shield against secondary injury in the spinal cord, at least in some animals."

Electrical work with nerves is much more speculative than the work being done with bones, Dr. Cohen emphasizes. But, he says, "I wouldn't be at all surprised if one day there were a machine that could deliver electricity to heal nerves just as there is now one that can heal bones."

Regenerating Arms and Legs

And if nerves can be regrown, why not limbs? It's a mind-boggling notion, but one for which researchers have hope, however reserved.

Animals like the salamander depend on electrical stimulation from nerves to regenerate lost limbs. If enough of the nerves leading to the severed limb are removed, the limb won't grow back. But if nerves from another part of the salamander are then threaded to the stump of the severed limb, regeneration will occur. In the salamander, regeneration occurs because the cells in the stump of the lost limb have the ability to revert, or dedifferentiate, from their specialized state as muscle, bone or nerves. They become primitive, embryoniclike cells, Dr. Becker explains. It's this tissue that reorganizes and grows into a perfectly formed salamander leg or tail, all apparently under the direction of naturally occurring electrical currents.

In humans, only certain cells found in the bone marrow are known to naturally dedifferentiate. These cells start the process of fracture healing by reverting to the kind of primitive, bone-building cells seen in infants.

But some researchers, including Drs. Becker and Bassett, think other cells also have the ability to revert to a primitive state and regrow lost arms or legs. What they don't have is the natural stimulus to do so—the electrical connection. And that's something they believe could be added. Far out? Perhaps. But electrical stimulation has been used, although not entirely successfully, to regenerate limbs in rats and frogs which would not normally have this ability.

"Certainly there is increasing evidence that the regeneration of limbs and spinal cords in animals that normally regenerate is being directed by electrical events in that animal," Dr. Bassett says. "If we can begin to define what normally occurs in the regenerating process, and mimic those same kinds of electrical environments in nonregenerating animals, it's entirely conceivable that we can make them, too, regenerate limbs. There is enough information now for us to say that one day we will understand it, and perhaps even be able to do it in mammals, including man."

Something Old, Something New

The use of electricity in medicine is nothing new. Two thousand years ago, Roman physicians used electric eels to ease the pain of gout-swollen feet. And devices very similar to those used today to heal bones were popular as long as 80 years ago, Dr. Bassett says. "The problem then, and what threatens to be a problem now, is that electricity is on the verge of being abused by people who will not put in the laboratory work to verify a product's effectiveness before offering it for clinical use."

He has a reminder of that in his office. It's a contraption one of his patients found in his grandmother's attic. You insert electrode A into your mouth, electrode B into your anus, set the dial on circuit five, and voilà, your hemorrhoids (and probably your halitosis, too) are supposedly cured.

If it's exploited this way, the whole field of bioelectricity could be labeled quackery, Dr. Becker says. "But if it's done properly, it will revolutionize the practice of medicine in the next two decades."

Stress Control Reports

Stress Patrol: How to Spot a Sneak Attack

So you've taken a personal inventory and decided that you're doing just fine in the battle against stress—no ulcers, no migraine headaches, no heart problems or hypertension, just the usual little physical and mental inconveniences that come with life: a rash, muscle aches every now and then, a touch of constipation, more problems with colds and flu than normal, and maybe forgetfulness and frustration at times. But stress? No problem.

Perhaps you shouldn't strain your arm patting yourself on the back. These minor conditions that are so easily ignored or attributed to other causes may in fact be warning signs that stress is nibbling away at you physically and mentally. If unchecked, a recurring combination of these innocent-looking conditions could in the short term most certainly affect the way you think and feel, and in the long term possibly lead to more traumatic problems, such as ulcers, a heart condition or hypertension.

"About 8 million Americans have ulcers, or at least that's how many we know about, but there are far more people out there suffering from these minor signs of stress who don't realize it," says Edward Charlesworth, Ph.D., a Houston psychologist and coauthor of *Stress Management: A Comprehensive Guide to Wellness* (Atheneum, 1984).

Ignorance Isn't Bliss

There are two consensus theories about why most of these minor signs of stress go unnoticed: Most people have no idea that these common, everyday maladies and behavioral quirks could be stress related; and we have become a nation that seems to take pride in denying that something is wrong.

"When you ask people about physical problems associated with stress, most automatically mention heachaches," says Mark McKinney, Ph.D., a psychologist in the department of preventive and stress medicine, University of Nebraska, Omaha. "People don't relate stress to minor symptoms, such as waking at 3:00 A.M. every day and having trouble falling asleep, or having too many colds. Or they may be working just as hard, and organizing their day but not getting as much done. They don't associate that with stress either."

Paul Rosch, M.D., president of the American Institute of Stress, Yonkers, New York, says he sees too many people who believe physical and mental problems are "the norm." "People often think they're supposed to have headaches, back problems, muscular aches and depression," Dr. Rosch says. "They accept these conditions as part of life in the twentieth century."

A stress specialist who spends his days helping people cope with the pressures of New York City had a firsthand lesson early in his career about the effects of stress. After leaving a small town for life in the big city, Howard Shapiro, M.D., fell in love with a house that he just had to have, even though it was a bit too expensive. Shortly after deciding to buy his dream home his stomach began to feel queasy, his appetite decreased and his thoughts were foggy at times. One day he went to a movie with friends and for a few hours, lost himself in cinematic make-believe, during which time his strange feelings vanished. Shortly after leaving the theater the uncomfortableness returned.

"While I was watching the movie, I was able to relax and concentrate on something that was totally make-believe." He says, "When it was over and my thoughts returned to the real world, my subconscious started letting me know that deep down inside I wasn't too comfortable with the obligation and financial commitment I was about to make.

"I use this example with many of my stress-management patients because when people don't feel well they look for major physical problems. The cause of their discomfort may be subtle and unobvious on the surface, however, and once they realize this, their physical conditions improve." He eventually decided not to buy the house.

Sound familiar? Probably. Consider the following groups of fairly common conditions that you may know all too well:

Off the Tract

Diarrhea, constipation and flatulence are usually attributed to "something I ate" and rarely to stress, but any of these three conditions, in combination with other symptoms, often indicates stress, says Dr. Charlesworth. When a 42-year-old woman came to his office complaining of diarrhea, depression, anxiety, sweating and palpitations, further tests revealed the suspected stress, and also a floppy heart valve.

"In this case we were looking for sources of stress and were able to catch the physical problem as well."

There's a Bug Going Around

As a college undergraduate, Dr. Charlesworth was constantly faced with yet another paper due in a week or a test next Friday. His health always managed to hold up during the days before the assignments were due. But as soon as the paper or test was completed and he was primed for a break, a cold or flu always got in the way.

"The strain had depleted my resistance abilities. My system managed to hold out just long enough so I could do the work, then I'd get sick when it was over because my immunity was low. I used to load up on vitamins but that made no difference," he says.

Colds, flu and allergic reactions are common, but if you have more than before, the reason could be stress. "If you tax the immune system long enough it will eventually fail, and chances are that you won't have the ability to handle the big problems when they come along," says Dr. McKinney.

"I Knew It Just a Minute Ago"

No one remembers everything, but forgetting a phone number that you use fairly often, daydreaming excessively or lapsing in concentration may be minor symptoms of stress. A young Louisiana woman who learned relaxation techniques to help cope with other problems in her life found that her concentration improved to the point that she was able to read a book, a task that previously had been impossible.

"Anxiety and stress interfere with the ability to learn and recall, and people who take relaxation training say it sharpens their memories," says Ronald Nathan, Ph.D., of the departments of psychiatry and family medicine at Louisiana State University Medical School, Shreveport, and coauthor of *Stress Management: A Comprehensive Guide to Wellness.*

The most common examples of forgetting under stress come when a student holds test in hand and can't remember a bit of the information that he has been studying the past five days, or upon reaching the podium a speaker's mind is suddenly blank.

Sweet Dreams Turn Sour

She was an English teacher, a perfectionist who was highly rated by her students and head of the department. During the summer months she slept like a baby, but when the school bells rang her slumbers were less than golden. She slept fine all through the night on Friday and Saturday, but she barely closed her eyes after the sun set on Sundays, and it wasn't much better Monday through Thursday.

"The stress of getting up and facing another day at school was manifesting itself in her sleep patterns," says Dr. Charlesworth. "She was fine on the weekends."

A bed is supposed to be for relaxation, but experts report that it can be an intense place for many people. Common problems include difficulty falling or staying asleep, waking at

3:00 A.M. and being unable to fall back asleep, insomnia and decreased sex drive, all of which can be stress induced.

Under the Skin

An astute teenager with a keen sense of deduction will tell you that more acne pimples pop out the day before a big date than after eating chocolate. Some people are genetically predisposed to skin problems, but acne, rashes and hives are often triggered or aggravated by stress, says Dr. Charlesworth.

Dermatologists have also linked eczema and dermatitis to stress, and a correlation has been drawn to hair loss, as several Houston teenagers found when the strain of wanting to get ahead and be the best took its toll on their scalps. There were probably telltale signs in the early stages that could have warned of too much stress, says Dr. Charlesworth, who has been involved with several of these unrelated cases, but the stress on these achievement-oriented teenagers went unchecked until bald patches were noticed.

Weak-Link Theory

One of the most baffling pieces in the stress puzzle is why some people experience a neck ache or decreased sex drive, while others may stutter slightly or have trouble concentrating. The most popular theory points to genetics.

"The body breaks down where it's the weakest, so a weak link in the family history may help determine where stress will show itself," says Dr. Nathan. "If the parents had hypertension or back problems or were prone to muscle-tension headaches, the chances are the offspring will have similar problems."

As a child, a person might have suffered a physical or emotional trauma that could have weakened the body, which could predispose that person to stress-related disorders in that weakened area, he says.

Almost half the United States population is ripe for back and muscle problems, says Lyle Miller, Ph.D., a clinical psychologist specializing in stress research at Boston University Medical Center. "About 40 percent of the population has one

MINOR SYMPTOMS
THAT MAY SIGNAL STRESS

If you check a significant number of items in this list, you may want to evaluate the stress in your life. Remember: What may be a symptom of stress in one person could be nothing more than a normal reaction for someone else.

☐ rashes
☐ more colds than normal
☐ hives
☐ memory slips
☐ concentration slides
☐ foot or finger tapping
☐ teeth gnashing, grinding
☐ awaking at 3:00 A.M. and being unable to fall back asleep
☐ appetite disorders (eating too much or losing appetite)
☐ diarrhea
☐ heart palpitations
☐ eyelid twitching
☐ difficulty falling or staying asleep
☐ minor back pain
☐ sudden bursts of energy
☐ increased sweating
☐ more minor accidents than normal
☐ flatulence
☐ frowning/wrinkled forehead
☐ feelings of suspiciousness, worthlessness, inadequacy or rejection
☐ anticipating the worst

leg slightly shorter than the other, so these people are automatically susceptible to back problems if stressed."

Your Body Barometer

A weak link could be used as a stress barometer, says Dr. Nathan. For example, a person prone to minor backaches could take preventive measures at the first sign of lower back discomfort, and possibly avert more serious problems.

The best way to recognize that stress is influencing your life is through personal awareness, the experts agree.

"It's similar to knowing when something's wrong with your car," says Dr. Charlesworth. "If you drive it every day, you know when it doesn't sound right or if there's a strange ping. If

MINOR SYMPTOMS
THAT MAY SIGNAL STRESS
—*Continued*

- [ ] nervousness before anything happens
- [ ] not recognizing a personality shift and refusing to believe it when pointed out
- [ ] cold hands or feet
- [ ] halitosis
- [ ] rapid heartbeat
- [ ] racing thoughts
- [ ] feeling trapped
- [ ] anger, irritation
- [ ] feeling that things are getting out of control
- [ ] muscle aches
- [ ] allergies
- [ ] jaw pain
- [ ] minor stomach discomfort
- [ ] bloated, full feeling
- [ ] constipation
- [ ] facial tics, twitches
- [ ] slight stutter
- [ ] dry mouth
- [ ] difficulty swallowing
- [ ] nausea, vomiting
- [ ] chronic fatigue
- [ ] lack of interest in sex
- [ ] gaining/losing weight
- [ ] menstrual distress
- [ ] cold, clammy hands
- [ ] frequent bouts with flu
- [ ] arthritic joint pain
- [ ] indecisiveness
- [ ] frustration
- [ ] anxiety, panic

we study our bodies, we'll be able to tell when something's wrong. We're constantly driving ourselves too hard and not noticing the little things our bodies are telling us.

"It's as simple as watching an exciting movie and noting how your body responds to excitement and tension. Then the next time your body is tense or excited, you'll be familiar with the feelings."

A change in attitude is also in order, Dr. Nathan says. "People don't view stress as a problem. If there's no physical sign, like stomach pain or an ulcer, they don't realize these little symptoms are telling them that corrective action is needed."

Above all, get to the root of the problem, stresses Dr. McKinney. Don't just cure the rash or constipation without also considering the stress that could have originally triggered the bodily reactions.

"All you have to invest is a little time. I've never seen anyone waste time learning how to detect and handle stress," he says. "It's like buying an appliance. How much you know can only help you."

Dr. McKinney labels it a consumer issue. "In this case especially, people need to be more responsible for their own health and not leave it in the hands of their physician. The medical community has its hands full curing problems that already exist and doesn't spend much time focusing on prevention."

It also helps to keep an eye on those around you, says Dr. Miller. "When you notice a friend or relative displaying some of these minor signs, tell them. They'll probably bite your head off and tell you to mind your own business, but you'll be doing them a favor in the long run. Wouldn't you want someone to tell *you*?"

If you have only two or three minor stress symptoms, chances are that you're in good shape. Even if you have a combination of symptoms, the experts caution that you shouldn't automatically conclude that an ulcer or heart attack is right around the corner.

There's also the possibility that the symptoms may not be stress related at all. "Diet, hormonal imbalances and other physiological problems can wear the mask of stress or anxiety symptoms," Dr. Charlesworth cautions.

Corrective Action

Once your awareness has been sharpened and you can spot the minor symptoms of stress, the corrective measures are the same as those used for coping with migraines, ulcers, heart attacks and hypertension: relaxation techniques, exercise, stress-management procedures and changes in diet.

Time management is another good coping technique, says Dr. Nathan. "People need to establish priorities and set realistic goals. Many of us spend more time planning parties than we do planning our lives.

"But you need to do all of this gradually, and don't get sucked up in the four-day phenomenon, which is very common when people try to make changes in their lives. They're so determined that they diet to starvation and exercise to exhaustion. Then they give up and go back to their old habits."

Adds Dr. Charlesworth, "Ninety-five percent of the U.S. population would benefit from some sort of stress-management training. We need to break the stress spiral by starting with these minor symptoms."

First Aid for Your Feelings

At some time in their lives, everyone suffers the type of emotional wound that can take months or years to heal. The loss of a friend, the death of a loved one or a divorce all modify life in far reaching and unalterable ways.

The vast majority of life's emotional hurts, though, are little ones—the garden-variety upsets that can leave you rattled for a day or two. Still, who wants to waste even one day on negative emotions? And the more hassles we have to deal with, it seems, the more disturbed we are likely to be by the *next* little incident that comes along.

How can you stop those emotional cuts and scrapes from turning into a major malady? By stocking your mental medicine chest with a handy supply of Band-Aids for the soul.

We've compiled a list of some typical, everyday upsets, and asked psychologists for their tips on how to make a quick recovery. Their suggestions are specific, but the underlying principles can be applied to most of the common hassles you might encounter.

For example, when you get caught at a traffic light, does your face turn red?

"There are three general strategies for dealing with that type of situation," says Robert D. Kerns, Jr., Ph.D., assistant clinical professor of psychology in psychiatry at the Yale University School of Medicine. "The first is behavioral—*doing* something to minimize the frustration. If you're caught at a traffic light, for instance, you can turn on the radio to distract yourself, or roll down the window to get a breath of fresh air.

"The second type of strategy is called cognitive, and

refers to what you *think*. For example, tell yourself positive statements. If you're late for an appointment and get caught in a traffic light, you can tell yourself, 'I'll make it, it's only one light, it only lasts 60 seconds.' You can even count the seconds.

"Another cognitive strategy is to distract yourself by thinking about a different, more pleasant scene. You can imagine what you'll do to relax at the end of the day, or imagine walking in your yard, looking at the garden."

If you really are going to be late, you might want to take a slightly different approach. "In that case, it's probably not the traffic jam that's causing you distress, but anticipation that something awful or catastrophic will happen later because of being late," says Dr. Kerns, who is also chief of the counseling and health psychology section at the Veterans Administration Medical Center in West Haven, Connecticut. "Rehearsing how you're going to cope with that future situation is a positive way to distract yourself. You might decide to make a joke about catching every light, make a simple apology, or just be ready to get down to business when you do arrive. That's a useful way to spend that time.

"The third strategy is to use relaxation techniques to minimize your emotional distress or the physiological arousal associated with it. Sit comfortably in your seat and relax all of your muscles very quickly until you become like a rag doll, or close your eyes for 15 seconds."

The Left-Out Feeling

Have your friends ever forgotten to invite you to an outing? Have you every had a birthday that nobody remembered? Or has your son or daughter ever forgotten to send you a card on Mother's Day?

"It's important to recognize that at one time or another everyone has forgotten a date, forgotten to send a card or to call," says C. Eugene Walker, Ph.D., professor of psychology at the University of Oklahoma College of Medicine in Oklahoma City and author of *Learn to Relax* (Prentice-Hall). "We all fall down. There probably isn't a person who hasn't done it or had it happen to him. You have to realize that it's just a part of life."

"It's not the fact that you didn't get the card that's so upsetting," Dr. Kerns told us, "but the negative thinking that goes along with it. A person prone to become distressed by those situations will go into a whole internal tirade about the event—all of the awful things that are meant by it. They'll say, 'This means they don't think of me, don't care about me, don't love me.' They'll think back to similar situations in the past that brought about similar feelings and they'll dwell on them. Psychologists refer to that type of thinking as negative cognitive distortion. It's common in people with depression.

"The strategy for dealing with that is to catch yourself early on in the phase of negative thinking and try to stop it," Dr. Kerns says. "Not by saying, 'Don't think that,' because as soon as you say, 'Don't think about X,' you're going to think about X more and more. What you really want to do is think of positive statements—a different way of evaluating the same situation. You can say, 'Maybe the card is late. I've sent late cards before. I can probably expect it later in the week. And if I don't get one, it's not the end of the world.' The idea is to minimize negative thinking by thinking more rational thoughts."

Overload

When your schedule has you swamped and you're ready to set fire to your office, you can use these pointers to get you back on an even keel.

"First, you need to be realistic about what you can get done," says Robert Felner, Ph.D., director of training in clinical psychology at Auburn University. "Don't say 'I'll work 40 hours straight and finish everything.'

"One of the best ways to approach a work overload is to map out exactly what you've got to get done and prioritize the list. There's no way to deal with a general work overload, but you can deal with each of ten tasks individually. That way, at the end of the day you can look at what you've accomplished instead of feeling like you've failed. There are too many people who spend a day being very productive and go home feeling like they didn't get anything done because everything isn't finished."

"Schedule in breaks—periods of reward to gather each

step along the way," suggests Dr. Kerns. "Tell yourself that you will make it through. Appreciate that you've made it through similar situations before and that you'll do it again."

Marital Spat

If a fight with your spouse ruffles your feathers for a whole day, you may want to learn some strategies for smoothing things out more quickly.

"I can really be affected by marital spats," says Stephen D. Fabick, Ed.D., a clinical psychologist from Birmingham, Michigan. "One thing that helps me is just realizing that it's going to happen every so often. You can't have your happiness totally dependent on whether you and your spouse are getting along that day. And you can't judge your relationship by it either."

"It's important to make plans for solving the problem," says Dr. Walker. "It's very disturbing to leave a problem open or unsettled. Propose a strategy and make a date to discuss it later." That way, it's easier to get on with your day.

"You might want to plan to do something special when you get home to make up," says Dr. Kerns. "That's a more positive way to think about it."

Butterflies

Most people are familiar with that fluttery feeling they get in their stomachs when they have to give a speech, take a test, or go to a party at the boss's house. That feeling is often more distressing than the actual event.

"That's referred to as anticipatory anxiety," explains Dr. Kerns. "It's not so much the doing of the task that's so anxiety producing, but the anticipation of it—the ruminating about it. We tend to think about the event in ways that provoke intense anxiety. The result is butterflies in the stomach, a headache or other symptoms.

"A good strategy is to realize that you are responsible for what you're doing to yourself, and that you have the ability to control those feelings," he says. "You can say, 'It's not the situation—it's my thinking about it that's generating the anxiety. I'm responsible, I'm in control and I'm able to do something about it.'

"If it's a speech you're giving, you can organize your talk and practice it. If it's a social engagement you're dreading, you can think about who'll be there, and mentally rehearse what you might say to them.

"You can also use relaxation techniques," recommends Dr. Kerns. "They'll reinforce your feeling of control because you'll see that you have the ability to do something. But there's also a physiological rationale for doing them. They literally loosen your muscles, slow your heart rate, and control your blood pressure."

The most widely prescribed relaxation technique is progressive muscle relaxation. You do it by systematically tensing and relaxing the various muscle groups in your body to generate a sense of total body relaxation. Deep, regular diaphragmatic breathing can also help you relax. The shallow chest breathing we do most of the time seems to go along with anxiety.

Another good relaxation technique is called positive imagery. That's where you imagine a relaxing scene, using as many senses as possible. "A beach scene works well for me," Dr. Kerns told us. "I imagine being alone on the beach, watching the waves rippling, hearing the sound of the waves breaking on the shore, tasting a hint of salt in the air and feeling the warm sun and sand. Some people like to imagine walking through the woods on a crisp fall day. For others, sitting in a rowboat on a lake with a fishing line is very relaxing. Whatever your scene is, the more elaborate and detailed you make it, the more relaxing it will be."

"You should also recognize that anxiety is part of life," says Dr. Walker. "That's much less upsetting than having the attitude that it's terrible and you shouldn't have to feel it."

In fact, you may even be able to put that anxiety to good use. "Up to a point, anxiety can really help people," says Dr. Fabick. "If we realize that, we can use it to our advantage. Many actors and actresses say that they get nervous, but it helps them get up for the performance. If you accept the normalcy of the anxiety and harness the energy in a positive way, it can help you."

Big Plans Fall Through

Have you ever looked forward to something, like a vacation or a visit with your family, and had it fall through at the last minute? Maybe you were planning for it, dreaming about it, and when it fell through it left you feeling a little blue.

"It's important to realize how understandable it is that you would feel disappointed," says Dr. Kerns. "You don't want to cover it up with Pollyannaish statements. But it's also important to put it in perspective."

"You can do things to be good to yourself to reduce the disappointment," suggests Dr. Felner. "Try doing a couple of little things that are fun. Sometimes people punish themselves after a disappointment and don't do anything. That just makes things worse. You can say, 'Gee, I won't get to go to the Bahamas this year but I can take a couple of side trips. And there are a lot of fun and productive things that I can do around here.'"

"It's great to get excited," says Dr. Fabick. "But with any expectations you've got to keep in mind that you can't count on things always working out. You don't want to go to the other extreme, though, where you never get excited about anything. The healthiest people seem to be able to find some balance of realistic expectations, keeping in mind that Murphy's Law is always operating ['If anything can go wrong, it will'].

"Another preventive measure is having several options. Many times we become so focused on just one possibility that if it falls through we become despondent."

Long-Distance Family Fight

With family members already living in distant places, a fight can make you feel light-years apart. And feeling cut off from your loved ones can be terribly distressing.

"The first thing to do is take a breather," says Dr. Kerns. "Take a brief period of time to cool off. But the bottom line is to reestablish contact soon. The worst thing is to avoid further contact with the person. That only potentiates the feelings of guilt, sadness, anger and distrust. Reviewing the fight in your mind will also amplify the distress you're feeling, and make you more likely to avoid a person that you care about. When you keep in contact, though, there's always the possibility of working things out."

"Be active at problem solving rather than letting things sit and fester," agrees Dr. Felner.

"Think through what has happened, how you would want it to come out and what you can do to remedy the situation," he suggests. "You can seek support from friends to calm yourself and get ideas."

You've Lost Your Temper

Have you ever gotten so angry that you've felt dangerous? Or has one of your outbursts left you feeling shaken, scared or even guilty?

First off, step back. "Instead of trying to justify your anger, take steps to reduce it," suggests Dr. Felner. "Don't act on that anger. Instead, sit down, take deep breaths and try to relax. Most people find that when involved in an argument, if they can get out of the same room for 15 minutes they're okay. They just need that time to pull back and calm themselves."

"It's a good idea to discharge the energy physically by taking a brisk walk or by participating in some other form of exercise," says Dr. Fabick. "And realize that it's normal sometimes to want to choke somebody. Don't feel guilty about it, just don't do it."

Teenage Tussle

Anyone who's lived with a teenager probably knows what life on a roller coaster is like. One minute everything's fine and the next minute your child is screaming, "I hate you!" Maybe you even scream back.

"At times like those, your strongest link is with the other parent," says Dr. Kerns. "It's important to reach out to that person for support and to align with them.

"The pain you can feel in that situation is not simple to deal with. You might be able to minimize it, though. If you know full well it's a temporary thing, tell yourself that. Don't overdramatize it—keep it in perspective. You can say, 'He's not lost forever, we'll get over it in the next few days.' You can see it as just one upset in a long line of events and seeming catastrophes in raising a child. It starts in infancy and continues all the way through."

"If *you've* gone overboard, acknowledge your own regret. And address it if the teen has, too," says Dr. Fabick. "Kids do well with parents who have the strength to admit mistakes."

Dr. Felner agrees. "It's unfortunate that parents have been fed all that stuff about consistency being more important than everything else. If you've lost your temper, you can apologize. Sometimes in a rage a parent might tell a kid that he's grounded for a month. If it's unreasonable, you can go back and say 'Look, I was angry and upset. I said the wrong thing. You're only grounded for two days. I'm sorry.' You'll both feel better."

A Brief Note of Caution: These suggestions are meant to help you keep your composure when faced with normal, everyday hassles. If any of these situations pose serious problems for you, you may also want to seek professional help.

Busy Person, Calm Mind

"I thought I was crazy," says Debra Kelly, a 34-year-old engineer and mother of two from Denver. "I could be at work, or home reading a book or taking a bath and suddenly I would have these feelings of absolute terror. Or I would wake up crying and shaking, and my heart would be skipping beats.

"I would get in the car to come to work and I would get lost on the way. And I was so claustrophobic that I would feel trapped at my desk if another person were sitting between me and the door. I had no appetite and was consuming nothing but coffee; I lost 25 pounds and looked like walking death.

"I went to an internist and he gave me a prescription for tranquilizers. I got so hooked I couldn't get off them."

Now, Debra, who is chief of product assurance for research and development at Martin Marietta Denver Aerospace, looks healthy, calm and self-assured. "When I learned how to relax myself, I got off the tranquilizers and the whole world changed," she says. "I felt like I was awake for the first time in two years. My appetite came back and I started gaining weight. Now I can go into a crowded office and it doesn't bother me the way it used to. My heart hasn't skipped a beat and I've had just one anxiety attack that I can remember in the last nine months."

Debra Kelly's story is not unusual. At least, not among the people who've gone through the stress-reduction program offered by the Human Performance Institute in Lakewood, Colorado, a suburb of Denver.

This innovative program, developed by clinical psychologist Michael Uhes, Ph.D., director of the Institute, is helping highly valued, hard-driving professionals gain control of the stress in their lives. And it is *making* money for the companies who pay for their employees to attend.

The Bottom Line

The program is packaged in a way that meets industry's needs. It has a beginning and an end (six to eight individual sessions with a therapist and three group sessions), a fixed cost ($585 to $650 per person) and it get results.

"Even if a company didn't care about its employees' blood pressure, sleeping problems or mental clarity—if all it cared about was cutting time lost from work—the program more than pays for itself," says Dr. Uhes. "For every dollar a company invests in an employee, before the first year is over those dollars will be paid back. Before two years are up, it gets an equal amount back. That is an unbelievable incentive for industry."

The incentives for the employees are just as good.

In research by Dr. Uhes and his staff, the numbers speak clearly. After participating in Dr. Uhes's four-month stress-reduction program, the frequency of headaches in the 300 people studied was down 58 percent, insomnia was down 66 percent, indigestion was down 41 percent and low back pain was down 53 percent. Shoulder and neck pain went down 73 percent, chest pain (angina) 69 percent, and diastolic blood pressure dropped 12 points. Follow-up six months to two years later still showed significant drops. The figures for psychological changes were similar. The people felt more joyful, satisfied, clearheaded and tranquil, and less discouraged, angry, rushed, distracted and frustrated.

"It's generally recognized that people under stress don't work very well," says Edward Dash, Ed.D., manager of management development and training at Martin Marietta, which designs and assembles space and defense systems. "So the benefits are pretty obvious to us. Often these people are in senior positions in the company. If they have the ability to cope with stress, then we have a more productive employee. It's not just rhetoric."

Martin Marietta was the first company to implement Dr. Uhes's program, but a dozen companies in the Denver area now have agreements with the Institute.

Most people sign up for the program because they are experiencing stress-related physical symptoms. Many have high blood pressure that cannot be controlled by medication. Some have had heart attacks. Ulcers, colitis and irritable-bowel syndrome are the three main gastrointestinal complaints. Many have low back pain, neck and shoulder pain, coronary artery disease or insomnia.

But psychological symptoms are common, too. "People under a lot of stress start forgetting things, particularly things that just happened," says Dr. Uhes. "And their thinking is polyphasic or scattered. They want to do one thing, but it's as if it's beyond their control to stay focused."

Some people are just overwhelmed at work. "It's not unusual to have a 50-year-old weep from the pressure and frustration," says Dr. Uhes.

Achiever's Disease

Why do professionals or high achievers have such problems with stress? "I call them disorders of the conscientious," says Dr. Uhes. "These people put too much pressure on themselves to do a good job at work. They face short deadlines. And they get a lot of frightening messages. They hear that there's a shakeup at corporate headquarters, for example. What can the average employee do about it except fret and worry?"

High achievers tend to be overscheduled in their work as

well as in their personal life. "Relaxation? It never occurs to them," says Dr. Uhes. "They don't know what relaxing means. They have little capability in that arena. They have often lost touch with the whole idea of taking care of themselves.

"These are not people who would normally go to a psychologist or psychiatrist. They are not mentally ill. They're very bright, they had excellent grades in college, they have wonderful families, successful marriages and they've done very well in their jobs. But their bodies start to come apart."

But most of the people who follow Dr. Uhes's program are finding relief. The program applies accepted techniques for stress reduction. It's different from other programs used by industry, though, because it's one-on-one, tailored for the individual and focused on changing that one person's life.

Getting Stress's Number

During the first session, the clients are taught how to quantify their stress on a scale of zero to ten, with zero being inner peacefulness and tranquillity and and ten being wired, tense and panicky—the most frightened they've ever been. Then they're given little notebooks that fit in a purse or back pocket and are asked to start noting whenever their stress level changes.

"Most of us experience emotions as a steady-state phenomenon," says Dr. Uhes. "Life's going great or life's really rough lately. We tend to conceive of our own existence in those terms, and that's totally inaccurate. We're not steady-state creatures. We're changing all the time. These people know they're stressed but they don't know the specifics."

All of the remaining sessions start off with a review of their record keeping. "We just listen," says Dr. Uhes. "We don't editorialize or try to bring a lot of insight. We just let the weight of the evidence come through and slowly it does come through. For each change in stress level they note, they are instructed to ask two questions. The first is, 'Where were you?' The second is, 'What happened?' We have them paint a very thorough picture of just what's going on. Who said what? Did your level go up then? What happened next? What were you thinking?

"What starts to happen is that what was for them a steady-state phenomenon ('I'm really tense and upset') starts to gain predictability ('Sometimes I'm tense and upset and this is what happens. I see a certain person's face, I think these thoughts, my body feels this way'). This rather unknown and general phenomenon starts to become very known to them, predictable and, finally, controllable."

"I started feeling better after four or five sessions," says Larry Feick, a 39-year-old senior industrial engineer at Martin Marietta. "The record keeping forced me to be aware of changes in my anxiety level in the early stages, and to grasp the thought I was thinking when I noticed a change. It's usually a negative thought, such as 'This traffic is maddening.' I learned to talk back in a positive vein: 'That's absurd. It's only a temporary condition.'"

Overstimulated

From day one clients are told to cut out caffeine. "These people are terrific self-stimulators," says Dr. Uhes. "It's not unusual for them to drink 8 to 12 cups of coffee a day. We give them samples of decaffeinated coffee.

"A very common method of operation we'll see is the person who, after fasting all night, will get up in the morning and have three cups of coffee, a couple of sweet rolls and a couple of cigarettes. Psychologically, that's a recipe for feeling anxious. Many of these people do not eat breakfast at all, or they'll eat while they're working at their desk. We insist they stop that. No more eating at your desk, no more talking about work while you eat. And we try to get them on something fairly close to a hypoglycemic diet: Get protein in the morning, don't skip any meals, and don't eat large amounts of simple sugar, particularly if that's all you're eating."

Exercise is an important component of the program, too. "If I had five minutes to talk to somebody about stress reduction, daily exercise would be the first thing I would suggest," says Suzette Cowles, R.N., one of the program's staff. "I've seen how people respond to it. They feel better and the world looks better when they exercise."

"We spend a lot of time helping each person find something they can do that they enjoy and that will be aerobic," says Dr. Uhes.

Because anxiety is a physical phenomenon as well as an emotional one, clients are also taught how to control their own physiological response to stress and thereby influence how they feel. "We make a cassette for them and ask them to play it once a day and practice the skills," Dr. Uhes told us. "We plop them down in a very comfortable chair and take them through all the muscle groups in the body and have them relax them, especially the musculature of the face. We could hand them a prerecorded tape, but we prefer to make one just for them, timed to their respiration. That's much more effective."

"The most helpful thing for me has been gaining the ability to systematically relax," says Patrick M Carter, a 48-year-old manager in the systems-engineering division of Public Service Company of Colorado. "When I began the program, my blood pressure was 135/103 and my doctor wanted to put me on medication. I don't smoke, I jog every day, I've watched my salt intake for years and I'm not overweight. I was already doing all the obvious things. When I finished the program my blood pressure was 107/75. It takes effort but it's ten times better than taking a pill for the rest of my life."

In a subsequent session, clients are given a more advanced relaxation tape. "Once they're in a calm state, we have them make some statements to themselves," says Dr. Uhes. "One we'll frequently have is, 'I am completely calm.' Another is, 'Move slowly, think slowly.' When people become stressed, everything speeds up—their thinking, their talking, their body processes—much to the detriment of their performance. In ensuing weeks, people will report that these thoughts are coming to them when they need them."

Honing Skills

As the program progresses, clients hone their relaxation skills even further. "They've been practicing relaxation every day using a 20-minute cassette," says Dr. Uhes. "Now we get them practicing doing the same thing very quickly, without a cassette. We call it the countdown technique."

The technique is based on breath meditation and takes

about five minutes. To do it, clients close their eyes, breathe comfortably, focus on the air coming in, and focus on the number five as the air goes out. After a couple of respirations, they let the number drop to four, and so on until they land on one. They focus on one for about a minute, then make the same statements to themselves as they did on the second tape. They focus on their breathing for another minute, then count themselves back up to five.

"They're taking a fragile skill that had to be practiced under optimum conditions and learning how to use it when they're 'in the frying pan,' rather than when they're at home lying in a recliner," explains Dody Schwartz, M.S.W., another of the program staff.

"We also describe ways to use the countdown technique like a 'stress inoculation' before going into a high-demand situation, such as a salary review," says Dr. Uhes.

Duane Tinnes, a 49-year-old chief of quality assurance at Martin Marietta and victim of a recent heart attack, found the countdown technique to be the most helpful thing he learned. "If someone was very demanding, I used to go into a high-tension state," he told us. "Now I count myself down and don't get excited. Someone can holler as much as they want to, it doesn't emotionally involve me. I could just about go to sleep in the middle of an argument."

Learning to Cope

In subsequent tapes, clients rehearse coping skills. "In a calm state, we have them image up the difficult situations, see and feel the beginning of their stress response, and picture themselves switching to a low-stress, coping response, feeling calm and thinking very clearly," says Dr. Uhes.

About six months after the final session, there is a follow-up questionnaire. And of course if they get into trouble, they know where to go for help. "Dr. Uhes says to call if I have a problem," says Bob Kessler, manager of Peacekeeper Weapon Systems Analysis at Martin Marietta. "If my blood pressure starts to go up, I'll see him again. But I don't think I'll need to. The tools he's given me are sufficient to deal with the world."

A Gun Called Stress

Can a piece of paper and a paper bag be considered instruments of death?

That's what a Maryland prosecuting attorney asked noted cardiologist and stress expert Robert Eliot, M.D.

The case involved a 60-year-old hotel desk clerk from Chevy Chase who was accosted late one night by two robbers. The two men handed her a note ordering her to put the contents of the cash drawer into the bag, promising "nobody will get hurt." But someone was. An hour and 40 minutes later, the woman dropped dead. Although there was no smoking gun, the prosecutor wanted to charge the two men with felony murder. He claimed they had frightened the clerk to death.

Dr. Eliot agreed to take a look at the evidence, in this case the coroner's sample of the woman's heart-muscle tissue.

"I had never seen such devastating changes in my life," says Dr. Eliot, director of preventive and rehabilitative cardiology at the Heart-Lung Center, St. Luke's Hospital, Phoenix.

The woman's coronary arteries were fairly clean, but her heart was riddled with lesions. "She had actually overdosed on her own adrenaline," says Dr. Eliot. "The answer to the question, can a piece of paper and a paper bag be instruments of death, is, unfortunately, yes."

After two days of deliberations, the jury concurred. It had indeed been murder by stress.

Though this was a legal milestone, the phenomenon of stress-produced sudden cardiac death is well known. In fact, stress can be what scientists call an "acute trigger" of sudden heart attack. It is one of six documented risk factors linked to heart attacks that occur "out of the blue." The others are snow (or extreme temperatures), Monday morning, recent consumption of a fatty meal, large consumption of alcohol and the hours between 6:00 A.M. and noon. Alone, or in combination, they can make an otherwise innocent day the perfect day for a heart attack.

Though, in some cases, the heart attack can occur in the absence of manifest heart disease, in the majority of instances

225

these triggers are a kind of last-straw assault on a cardiovascular system weakened by smoking, excess dietary fat and other factors.

Some heart attacks are linked to "sudden cardiac death," the leading cause of death in the United States. Most of its victims are men in their most productive years—their forties and fifties. One out of three has no apparent warning.

Though most have coronary artery disease or some other heart disease, a small percentage have no structural cardiovascular damage. The immediate cause of death is a heart arrhythmia called ventricular fibrillation, what one researcher describes as "an electrical storm" in the heart that causes it to pump erratically.

That is what killed the luckless hotel clerk—and, perhaps, her husband. "As an unfortunate consequence, he dropped dead two days before the verdict was reached," says Dr. Eliot.

Some of the most revealing research about the phenomenon is being done by scientists at Harvard and at Brigham and Women's Hospital in Boston. Four years ago, psychiatrist Peter Reich, M.D., and his colleagues made headlines when they found that a number of life-threatening ventricular arrhythmias were triggered by acute emotional stress—in one case, by something as minor as an exciting ball game.

The investigators questioned 117 survivors of these life-threatening arrhythmias—which are now survivable, thanks to modern emergency techniques. Twenty-five of these survivors had had acute psychological disturbances within 24 hours of the arrhythmia episodes. In 15 cases, the disturbances preceded the arrhythmia by only an hour.

One man, a 39-year-old ex-athlete, experienced irregular heartbeats when he grew violent toward his wife. In one case, a Yankees fan had ventricular fibrillation watching his team lose to the Red Sox on television.

None of the incidents that precipitated the arrhythmias were life threatening in themselves. In fact, they were only the trigger, not the bullet.

The bullet is the body's chemical response to acute stress. "Look on stress as the seventh-round knockout punch," says Dr. Eliot. "But you have six rounds of softening up."

The body's stress reaction was designed—quite cleverly actually—to prepare primitive man to survive encounters with a world that was truly out to get him. It produces chemicals that cause the blood pressure to rise, diverting blood from the skin and digestive organs to the muscles, which need to be strong to fight or flee. These chemicals also signal blood fats to flood the bloodstream for energy and the blood to clot quickly in case of injury.

Its response to chronic stress, on the other hand, stimulates the body to steel itself for the long wait under siege, which means conserving vital resources. That includes retaining water and salts, increasing gastric-acid production to make digestion more efficient, releasing high-energy fats and clotting agents into the bloodstream and slowly pushing up the blood pressure.

"This was a great thing when we were moving wagons across the prairies and looking for food and shelter, which is the way life was for millions of years," says Dr. Eliot. "Today, we engage this long-term survival reaction in our battles against invisible foes and unidentified problems. But, unlike millions of years ago, we have no relief. We've taught the brain to write the body a prescription that is an overdose of these stress chemicals. What was survival becomes suicidal."

What may be the most significant effect of this stress response is the damage it does to heart-muscle fibers. "It actually takes bites out of the heart muscle," says Dr. Eliot. "It can overcontract the small muscle fibers until some of them rip. This can produce electrical instability. The normal muscle fibers next to the dying fibers produce a chaotic electrical storm, which causes the heart to beat with a crazy rhythm. It then can't pump blood. And if it can't pump blood, you know the outcome.

"Now, you're saying to yourself, this can't be that common, can it? It's true in more than 84 percent of all victims of sudden death."

These harmful changes can occur even if blood cholesterol is normal and the arteries clean as a whistle, says Dr. Eliot. "What people need is emotional fitness," says the cardiologist, coauthor of the award-winning book *Is It Worth Dying For?* (Bantam, 1984), which outlines his stress-management techniques.

He developed those techniques during years of research

at the University of Nebraska, attempting to identify and help a specific group of people, whom he terms "hot reactors." These people, prime candidates for heart attacks, consistently have an excess cardiovascular response to stress.

Right now, Dr. Eliot's National Center of Preventive and Stress Medicine in Phoenix is attracting much attention because they identify potential heart-attack victims before the ultimate tip-off: the heart attack.

The underpinning of the program is self-assessment. For each person, a set of techniques (from exercise to attitude modification to relaxation) is prescribed, based on an individual evaluation of the stresses that are literally breaking their hearts. "The Germans have an expression, 'First the diagnosis, then the treatment,' " says Dr. Eliot. "It's not a bad idea. Once you know your stresses, you can put together a lot of different techniques to help you."

Blue Monday

In 1980, researchers at the University of Manitoba discovered a curious statistic: 75 percent of all sudden cardiac deaths occurred on Monday on the job.

Simon Rabkin, M.D., and his colleagues took a look at a grueling number of cases: 3,983 men who had been found fit for pilot training in World War II. They found that those who had obvious clinical signs of heart disease might be stricken at any time during the week. But those who did not almost always died suddenly on Monday at work. Also, almost half of those who died at home or other locations also died on Monday.

Why the preponderance of sudden deaths at work on Monday? According to the researchers' speculation, there may be more to the worker's traditional Monday morning blues than just grousing. "Reintroductions to occupational stress, activity or pollutants after a weekend respite may be factors precipitating the arrhythmias that are the presumed basis for sudden death," they conjectured. "Psychological stress has been related to sudden cardiac death and return to work may serve as a stressor" (*Journal of the American Medical Association,* September 19, 1980).

Oh, How I Hate to Get Up in the Morning

A Harvard researcher earlier this year discovered that heart attacks have their own apparent circadian rhythm. Most of the 847 cases cardiologist James E. Muller, M.D., studied occurred between 6:00 A.M. and noon. Dr. Muller, assistant professor of medicine at Harvard and a clinical cardiologist at Boston's Brigham and Women's Hospital, used information supplied by over 50 investigators nationwide to pinpoint the peak hours of myocardial infarction.

His findings confirmed the work of researchers in Europe, South Africa and the Soviet Union, who also found an early-morning heart-attack peak.

It's probably no coincidence that the 6:00 A.M.-to-noon period is also when heart rate, arterial pressure and physical activity also increase. Further study, Dr. Muller told a gathering of physicians at the American College of Cardiology in California last spring, "may help identify the events triggering MI [myocardial infarction] and present opportunities for primary prevention."

Baby, It's Cold Outside

Researchers—and hospital emergency-department personnel—have long known that heart attacks increase during snowstorms. "In New England, every time it snows we have a flood of heart attacks," says William Castelli, M.D., medical director of the famed Framingham Heart Study.

One speculation is that snow shoveling is the culprit. And it might well be in some cases. But some researchers suspect it may simply be the cold.

"In the lab, the effect of cold is well known," says Matthew Zack, M.D., of the chronic diseases division of the Centers for Disease Control, in Atlanta. "When people with angina pectoris are asked to exercise to the point where the pain begins, researchers find that these people cannot exert themselves as far—that is, walk as far or as fast—in a cold room as opposed to a warm room."

Dr. Zack and several of his colleagues were so interested in snow and cold as risk factors for heart attack, they undertook two studies (one following Chicago's 1979 blizzard) attempting to identify those people at high risk of snow-related myocardial infarction. They were unable to identify such high-risk people and they were also unable to pinpoint snow shoveling as the acute trigger of snowstorm heart attacks.

Exertion can bring on a heart attack, says the researcher, "but it could be just the cold. When you are cold, the blood vessels to the skin constrict so you can conserve body heat. Blood vessels to the heart may also constrict, cutting off the heart's blood supply. People with angina pectoris can increase the number of attacks and their severity just by exposure to cold. Of course, it doesn't always happen. It can happen in hot weather too. It's anything that causes the blood vessels to the heart to constrict. People with angina pectoris or arteriosclerosis usually have a fixed blockage. That doesn't change. But if you increase the work of the heart by constricting the vessels in another place, that may be enough to precipitate a heart attack."

The Last Supper

When researchers examined coroners' reports on 100 sudden deaths of British men listed as victims of coronary-artery disease, they found that about a quarter had died approximately an hour after eating. Although this particular investigation didn't turn up any significant link to the fat content of the men's last meal, there is other evidence that indicates that a high-fat meal can have devastating consequences on the cardiovascular system.

Investigators have found, for example, that blood fats, such as cholesterol and triglycerides, tend to increase; attacks of angina pectoris rise, as does platelet aggregation and clotting. Some people show changes in electrocardiograph readings that indicate a decrease in arterial blood flow. However, the entire cardiovascular system moves into high gear after a meal to help burn up the food as fuel.

Paul B. Roen, M.D., now retired senior director for the Clinic for the Study of Arteriosclerosis, in Los Angeles, once suggested that "heavy evening meal" be added to the risk factors for heart attacks and strokes. The peak of digestion, he notes, probably occurs during deep sleep periods when the body is unable to move blood fats through the arteries quickly. In arteries already damaged by atherosclerosis, he says, it's likely that those fats will be the insult added to injury, decreasing already narrowed arteries and providing an "ideal situation" for platelets to clot.

The same British researchers who examined coroners' reports on 100 sudden-death victims found that slightly less than a quarter had died shortly after consuming alcohol. In fact, investigators in Scotland, looking for acute triggers of sudden cardiac death, found that Saturday night and alcohol were the fatal combination. Other studies in this country have implicated binge drinking in sudden heart attack cases.

Apparently, for some vulnerable arteries, a drink on the wrong day is the ominous signal for closing time.

A Good Talk Is Good Medicine

● Three weeks after his grandfather dies of stomach cancer, a 12-year-old boy develops the same ominous pains. He and his parents are worried sick. Could he have cancer, too?

● A nine-year-old girl begins to have strange, seizurelike spasms in her arms and legs. A doctor at the hospital notes the girl's family is having a bitter argument. But each time the little girl breaks into one of her spells, they all stop fighting and rush together to her bedside.

● A teenager hasn't been to school for five years because he and his mother are convinced he's terribly ill. But dozens of sophisticated medical tests show nothing wrong, and the boy is growing normally. When the doctors suggest psychological counseling, the mother indignantly checks her son out of the hospital.

As these case histories illustrate, children are no more immune to stress-related illnesses than adults. In fact, they may be even more vulnerable. They have little control over their own lives, and may not have the language skills or self-confidence to say what's troubling them. If parents can't tune in to a child's way of thinking, and encourage him to express himself, they may miss the clues that indicate their child's illness is related to stress. And they also forfeit the chance to help their child learn healthy ways to handle feelings like fear, anger and hurt.

Like Father, Like Son

Pediatricians find that children frequently develop symptoms for which no physical cause can be discovered. One study of families of children with unexplained illnesses found a major family crisis in 97 percent, and a depressed parent in 85 percent. Sometimes, though, the illness is the result of smaller stresses that build up—family feuds, neighborhood bullies, failing grades.

It's not the stress itself, though, that causes the symptoms. It's the way the child reacts to stress that matters. And that's determined mostly by family behavior.

"Children who develop psychosomatic symptoms often come from upwardly mobile, striving, together kinds of families, at least on the surface," says Brian Stabler, Ph.D., associate professor of psychology and pediatrics at the University of North Carolina School of Medicine. But many of these families have trouble talking about problems.

"The family style may be to communicate more through physical complaints than through discussing what might make people feel uncomfortable," says Anthony Richtsmeier, M.D., assistant professor of pediatrics with the Chicago Medical School at Cook County Children's Hospital, Chicago. "A parent of a child with psychosomatic symptoms might say to her spouse, 'Not tonight, dear, I've got a headache,' rather than 'I'm just not in the mood, honey.' The child may learn to translate his anxieties over troubles at school or home into upset stomachs or headaches."

Pollyanna Outlook

Some of these parents seldom discuss unhappy events, Dr. Richtsmeier says. "They try to make the world look brighter than it is, rather than encourage the child to take his lumps, and adjust to the situation as best as he can. They are more likely to offer their children reassurance without helping them deal with their underlying anxieties. If their child is having trouble at school, instead of saying, 'I can sure understand why you are sad about what happened at school today. Would you like to tell me about it?' they'll say, 'Oh, don't worry about that,' or 'Everything will be okay.' "

The result is that their children become filled with conflict and confusion, Dr. Richtsmeier says. "They know they are still upset, but they're trying to put on a happy face. They feel compelled to keep tight lipped about feeling bad, and pretend that everything is fine when it isn't, and the tension, the energy this creates may develop into a physical symptom."

Dr. Richtsmeier found himself privy to what really bothers these children when he evaluated unexplained physical symptoms in youngsters who had been referred to him. He saw 24 children from 5 to 12 years old. All had persistent physical symptoms, such as stomach pains, headaches or limb aches. The symptoms had resulted in numerous medical evaluations and parental anxiety and had not responded to treatment in the past.

At the time the children were referred to him, all the families said they thought the symptoms had a physical cause. Asked directly, they said they did not think psychological causes had any major impact on the symptoms.

But that's not what Dr. Richtsmeier found when he interviewed each child alone. When they were asked specific questions about their relationship with parents, brothers and sisters, teachers and friends, and other questions such as what makes them happy or sad, and what worried them most about their symptoms, 18 of the children disclosed major sources of anxiety that had not been revealed in previous evaluations. And 14 said they suspected emotional factors had a direct influence on their symptoms. The primary reluctance or inability to face the emotional problem was often the parents', not the child's.

Asked to make three wishes, the children's answers were sometimes painfully touching. "I had children who said 'I wish Mom and Dad didn't fight so much,' 'I wish Aunt Susan was still alive,' 'I wish I had more friends,' " Dr. Richtsmeier says.

"The major worries for these children are parental relationships, separation from family, sickness and death, and being accepted into the outside world. The early school-age child has to get out and gain experience with his peers and autonomy from his family, and that's a difficult step for a lot of them. If it doesn't go well, and they're not being helped along the way by being able to talk about how to adjust, they'll have problems."

Allowed to discuss and resolve their anxieties, though, 15 of the 18 children in Dr. Richtsmeier's study found their symptoms quickly improved.

Childhood Misperceptions

Sometimes children will misperceive things. One little boy came to Dr. Richtsmeier with a strange case of amnesia. He had put his head down on his desk for a nap, and awakened not knowing who or where he was. "It turned out he had recently witnessed his aunt having a stroke, and his perception of it was that she didn't know who she was or where she was," Dr. Richtsmeier says. "As I talked to him, I found that he was worried he was going to have a stroke, too. In effect, he worried himself into the symptoms. As this child was helped to express his anxieties about his aunt's stroke, his symptoms abated."

And sometimes the child's symptoms serve a family purpose. The little girl with the strange twitching in her arms and legs had subconsciously discovered how to hold her family together. And her family's reaction reinforced her symptoms.

Grief into Pain

Often, these children are developing their first real understanding of mortality. "It's not unusual to find there has been an illness or death in the family recently," says Dr. Stabler, who treated the 12-year-old boy who developed stomach pains soon after his grandfather's death.

"Every case is different. That's why you have to find out about the child and his family before you can help. This boy's grandfather had been his only friend, and had taught him things on the farm. The grandfather's stomach cancer was diagnosed very late, and he had gone downhill quickly. This youngster never had the chance to resolve how great a loss that was to him. He was expressing his unresolved grief over his grandfather's death by psychologically identifying with him through symptoms."

The boy's parents were unaware of their child's distress. "The very nature of the psychosomatic problem implies that there is not an open discussion," Dr. Stabler says. "The pain represents everything. It was his loss, his sadness, his anguish, and words didn't need to be spoken. That's why, when you start to talk with a child like this, you need to listen a lot and put the pattern together."

Letting the boy talk about his grandfather helped him to feel some of his grief, Dr. Stabler says. "He cried, and that's okay for a little boy who is missing his grandfather."

Not "Playing Possum"

Moving from the physical to the emotional isn't easy, Dr. Stabler admits. "It's always a difficult transition, because the parents are very concerned that this is a real pain. It's absolutely vital to be clear that we are not saying this is a fake thing. This is not like a kid playing possum. A pain caused by stress is just as real as one caused by a physical condition. It's important to reassure parents of this, and emphasize it does not mean serious mental illness is involved."

In this case, for instance, Dr. Stabler says, "I told the parents that their son had a psychological pain that had converted to a physical pain. And they could understand that. They could understand how when things build up on you, you get a headache, how when you're nervous because you have to stand up in class, you get butterflies in the tummy. That helped them to focus concretely on how you can turn a feeling into a pain."

Dr. Stabler saw the boy weekly for about three months, until the pain resolved. He encouraged him and his parents to talk more. He also talked with the boy's teacher, so that there would be no more reinforcement of physical symptoms at school.

How Many Tests?

All the children Drs. Richtsmeier and Stabler saw had gone through extensive medical testing. One little girl had had her appendix removed in an attempt to relieve symptoms.

The 12-year-old boy had been seen by half a dozen different doctors in his area, and had finally been referred to the medical center, where Dr. Stabler worked with him as part of a pediatric-gastroenterology workup, including some major tests, like a colonoscopy.

Medical testing can be good and bad. Too many tests not only expose a child to unnecessary hazards, they can reinforce a family's conviction that their child has a terrible disease. But some medical evaluation is essential.

"Even if there's good reason to think your child's symptoms are stress-related, that doesn't mean there's not an underlying physical problem," says Dr. Richtsmeier. "There is no reason why physical and psychological problems can't coexist and interact with each other. It takes both the absence of a physical problem and the presence of a psychological one to make a psychosomatic diagnosis."

And the "cure" for psychosomatic symptoms requires that there be no lingering doubts that the doctor has overlooked something. "The family needs to be absolutely clear in their own minds that all possibility of cancer, tumor, ulcer or any other illness they might have considered has in fact been ruled out," says Dr. Stabler.

Just how many medical tests are done depends on the parents and doctor. Drs. Stabler and Richtsmeier suggest that it is often beneficial to explore emotional areas while continuing the evaluation for physical causes.

One rule of thumb might seem to be to do enough tests to satisfy both doctor and parent, but that doesn't always work. As in the case of the 17-year-old boy who hadn't been to school in five years, sometimes it's the very disturbed parent who insists on test after test, and who resists any psychological help.

What Can Parents Do?

Sometimes the tip-off for psychosomatic symptoms is obvious. "If a seven-year-old child gets a bellyache every schoolday morning and doesn't get one on weekends and the mother knows her kid is getting beat up in school, that's pretty clear," Dr. Richtsmeier says. Certainly, though, if there's any doubt whether the symptoms are stress related, a visit or call to the doctor is essential.

How parents react to their child's initial illness may determine whether the symptoms continue, Dr. Richtsmeier says. "Some can nip this right in the bud. Let's say they're at the dentist and their kid says he feels sick and wants to go home. If the child doesn't seem particularly ill they'll say, 'You're nervous about seeing the dentist, so it's not unusual for your stomach to be upset. But it's important for you to see the dentist, so we're not going to go home.' " Parents who cannot stand to see their child unhappy or frustrated, or who overemphasize the physical (always asking the child how he feels, for instance) reinforce their child's behavior.

You can't, and shouldn't, protect your child completely from stress, Dr. Stabler says. "I like the idea of what's known as psychological immunization. It means that during your child's early years you try to control the amount and type of stress the child has to deal with. In overcoming small, controlled stressors, like not getting everything they want or dealing with the death of a pet, kids psychologically become more capable of dealing with the larger stressors in life. The most successful parents are basically authoritarian, but willing to explain things to their children. They set rules, but they talk, too."

Being able to talk honestly and respectfully with your child is perhaps the best protection against psychosomatic ills. And it's a good idea to be aware of your children's perceptions of problems in the home, Dr. Richtsmeier says. "A good place to start is to ask them what they think. Don't just sit them down and give long explanations. Gear what you tell them to how old they are, and only tell them what they need to know. Be straightforward and clarify their misunderstandings. Let them know it is okay to ask questions."

Little bellyachers can grow into big bellyachers, Dr. Richtsmeier says. Helping your child overcome this behavior while he's young could avoid a lifelong problem.

Weight-Reduction Bulletins

Deficiencies That Hit Dieters below the Belt

Researchers have found that immune-system response drops in people on very-low-calorie diets, says Peter Lindner, M.D., director of continuing medical education for the American Society of Bariatric Physicians (obesity specialists). "In one study, the researchers were interested in the changes in disease-fighting white blood cells when exposed to vaccine. What they found was that the immune response was reduced in those individuals on improperly administered ultralow-calorie diets, making them more subject to infection. That is probably one of the most dangerous aspects of very-low-calorie diets."

If you're a dieter—and surveys show two out of three are—there's a very good chance you may be endangering your health, warns Dr. Lindner. You may be able to take nutrition for granted when you're eating like a horse, but it becomes critical when you start eating like a bird.

"A good balanced diet in the higher caloric range probably gives you all the vitamins and minerals you need. It gives you some leeway to play with," says the physician. "Drop it down to 800 or 1,000 calories and everything counts."

In fact, according to the Food and Nutrition Board of the National Academy of Sciences—which sets our Recommended Dietary Allowances—it is difficult to get adequate nutrition on diets that provide less than 1,800 to 2,000 calories. Most popular reducing diets call for 1,200 or less.

Balancing a Diet

It's hard enough to juggle the four food groups into a nutritionally balanced diet when you've got a few thousand calories to work with. Dieters have a tougher task. They have to concoct three healthful meals with roughly half the calories they're used to consuming. And they start out with a handicap—they don't know beans about nutrition.

Following a diet guide may not help. Many popular diet plans are full of dubious nutritional advice. And most dieters know only enough to plan a 1,200-calorie menu down to the last morsel. Knowing calories isn't enough. You can create three low-calorie meals a day without ever straying from the candy counter.

Perhaps the most important thing to remember when you're counting calories is that it's the nutitional value of the calorie that counts. If you don't know the value of a calorie, you don't know what you're missing.

But Paul LaChance, Ph.D., does. Dr. LaChance, professor of nutrition and food science at Rutgers University, evaluated the nutritional content of 11 published weight-loss diets. He chose the 11 because they ran the gamut of popular weight-reducing plans—from high-protein/low-carbohydrate to low-protein/high-carbohydrate, with variations in between. They carried such familiar names as Scarsdale, Stillman, Atkins and the Beverly Hills Diet.

Using the RDAs as a frame of reference, Dr. LaChance and associate, dietitian Michele C. Fisher, Ph.D., R.D., found that most of the diets were low in thiamine, vitamin B_6, vitamin B_{12}, calcium, iron, zinc and magnesium. Thiamine, vitamins B_6, and B_{12}, and magnesium were often at levels less than 70 percent of the RDA. One, the Beverly Hills Diet, supplied less than 70 percent of the RDAs for more than half of the vitamins and minerals they evaluated, and was so low in protein the researchers predicted it would lead to a serious protein deficiency over a long period of time.

And there's the rub. Most diets are protracted, if not forever. "Most people stay on a diet for a long time. After all, weight loss doesn't occur overnight," says Dr. LaChance. "If a diet lasts only two weeks, the vitamin and mineral loss is not going to be significant. As far as I'm concerned, women are dieting all the time and may have other risk factors—smoking, contraceptive-pill use—that can affect nutrient metabolism. For them, the loss can be very significant."

If fact, researchers studying otherwise healthy men found that even without those extra risk factors a prolonged low-calorie diet had a damaging effect on their health. One group, which had previously eaten over 3,000 calories daily, ate about half that for a period of six months. Even though they were eating more calories than prescribed by most reducing diets, the men suffered from depression, anemia, edema, slowing of heartbeat and loss of sex drive. They also tired easily and lacked endurance.

Some weight-loss regimens, specifically those that are mainly protein, can lead to a potentially serious condition called acidosis, which also can occur on fasting diets. In one study, people fed a diet of solely protein and fat lost about two pounds a day—along with large amounts of nitrogen and salt in their urine. They suffered from the symptoms of acidosis, which can include weakness, malaise, headache and heart arrhythmias.

Acidosis can be remedied by adding as little as about three ounces of carbohydrate to the diet.

Needless to say, bizarre diets that rely heavily on one food—such as grapefruit—are going to be nutritionally bankrupt. Very-low-calorie liquid diets can be deadly.

Women are always going to have to pay extra attention to the nutrient content of their diets because of their increased needs for certain nutrients. "For women it's hard enough to get things like calcium and iron." says Cindy Rubin, clinical nutritionist with the obesity research group at the University of Pennsylvania.

Women generally need more iron and calcium than men.

"Many women are going to have to supplement their diets with calcium and iron," says noted weight and fitness expert Gabe Mirkin, M.D., who ordinarily doesn't advocate dietary supplements. "One out of four women between 12 and 50 is iron deficient."

Though an iron deficiency may eventually lead to anemia, it has its own immediate health consequences. "When you're iron deficient, even though you're not anemic," says Dr. Mirkin, "you can't clear lactic acid as rapidly as normal from your bloodstream, so you tire easier at work and play."

"The problem with calcium is that it's scarce except in milk products—the first thing many dieters cut out. Unless you choose skim milk, dairy products can be high in fat and calories," says Dr. Lindner. "It's difficult to get adequate calcium without milk unless you want to eat sardines, small bones and all."

How food is prepared may also affect a dieter's nutrition. "If you're eating a salad that was tossed three days ago, vitamins are lost simply by exposure," says Dr. Lindner. "If food is cooked too much, you can lose more. Especially at risk are the water-soluble vitamins, such as C and B vitamins."

One of those B vitamins is folate. Women are particularly at risk of developing anemia when they aren't taking in enough folate, which is found in leafy greens. A form of anemia occurs when there isn't enough folate in the body to produce red blood cells. Folate deficiency also has been pinpointed as a factor in an often precancerous condition called cervical dysplasia.

Studies have also shown that low-calorie and starvation diets can lead to an excessive loss of zinc, possibly as a result of tissue breakdown. Researchers at the Veterans Administration Hospital in Hines, Illinois, found that weight-loss diets between 600 and 1,240 calories can be zinc deficient, depending on the type and source of dietary protein from which the zinc is derived. Diets that derive most of their protein from red meat tend to supply more zinc than those that rely on chicken, fish, milk products and eggs, which are, unfortunately, the main protein sources of many low-calorie diets.

If it all sounds discouraging, rest assured that the obesity experts understand—and have more than one solution to a dieter's nutritional dilemma.

● If you don't feel you can add red meat to your diet or if time and money constraints make it impossible to eat only freshly prepared foods, you can take supplements. "Theoretically, it's not necessary to supplement your diet," says Dr. Lindner, "but realistically most people don't have the knowledge or the time to do it right. Especially if you're a woman, a standard multiple vitamin that contains iron, B₆, folacin [folate] and zinc along with a calcium supplement should help you make sure you're getting all of the 26 micronutrients you need."

● Learn the value of a calorie. You know there's a big nutritional difference between a 200-calorie candy bar and a 200-calorie protein salad. But even so-called diet foods aren't created equal. "Choose nutrient-dense foods," suggests Cindy Rubin. "For instance, eat broccoli as opposed to lettuce. Both are low in calories, but lettuce is mainly water. You're not getting the heavy doses of vitamin A you get in broccoli."

● Go for variety. Not only is it the spice of life, it improves your chances of getting all the vitamins and minerals you need.

● Plan your diet menu from the four basic food groups. "Each of the major categories represents certain vitamins and minerals," says Dr. Mirkin. "Grains and cereals, for example, give you E and the B vitamins. Fruits and vegetables supply C and A. If you take in at least 1,500 calories a day and distribute your calories over the four food groups, you'll probably be taking in the nutrients you need."

● Eat more calories. We've saved the blockbuster for last. By eating more, naturally, you're more likely to meet your nutritional needs. But will you lose weight? Yes, say the experts, as long as you burn up some of those calories through exercise.

In his book *Getting Thin* (Little, Brown and Company, 1983), Dr. Mirkin advises eating 1,500 calories a day—and using an hour of exercise to burn off 300.

There are some unique advantages to this plan. Aside from losing weight healthfully, you'll stimulate your metabolism to burn even more calories. "You see, diets don't work," says Dr. Mirkin. "When you go on a diet, your metabolism slows down. When you're lying in bed, not even moving, you burn 60 calories an hour. If you're on a diet, you burn only 50. If you exercise, you burn 70—without even moving. Exercise speeds up your metabolism 24 hours a day, not to mention suppressing your appetite."

Dr. Mirkin recommends picking two sports—aerobic dancing and biking, for instance—and working up slowly to an hour of each on alternating days. "I specify two sports because it takes you 48 hours to recover so you should rotate the stressors on your body," he says.

Older people especially need exercise as an integral part of any diet plan. "The two have to be together," says Dr. LaChance. "When you're young, your metabolism is higher and you can get away with more. When you get older, your body changes. Your metabolism slows, your lean body mass goes down and your propensity for adipose [fat] tissue goes up. You lower your need for calories so if you don't add exercise, you get fat."

Trimming Down Junior

Baby fat is pinched, tickled, kootchykooed *and* grown out of, according to popular wisdom, which also considers it less harmful than diaper rash.

But last year, researchers in the nine-year-old Bogalusa Heart Study found that baby fat is far from benign. In fact, they warn, it may be an early warning marker of atherosclerosis, a time-bomb disease that begins as early as childhood and is responsible for one out of every two deaths in the United States.

The researchers, who published their findings in July, 1985, in the *Journal of the American Medical Association,* examined 1,598 children between 5 and 12 years old at five-year intervals. They discovered that childhood obesity was directly linked to increases in blood cholesterol, a fatty substance that clogs and damages the arteries.

Explains David Freedman, Ph.D., a member of the research team from the Louisiana State University Medical Center, "What we found was that the children gaining the most weight tended to have the largest increase in cholesterol levels, which led us to the conclusion that overweight is likely to be related to an increase in heart disease."

And statistically, it's the rare fat child who doesn't become a fat adult. Children often don't, as their mothers hope, "grow out of it."

Studies have shown that the longer a child is obese, the more likely he is to remain so. Only about 14 percent of all fat babies stay fat throughout their lives, but nearly three-quarters of all overweight teens become overweight adults.

Parents usually need little convincing that there's nothing pleasing about their child's plumpness—if they notice it at all. Unfortunately, parents are notoriously poor at judging whether Johnny is chubby. "They're with him every day," says James Sidbury, M.D., director of the program for obese children at the National Institute for Child Health and Human Development, in Bethesda, Maryland. "Usually the weight increases happen slowly. The thing that knocks them between the eyes is when the child goes from size XX to size XXX and they realize they can't put clothes on him anymore."

A pediatrician can provide a more objective judgment by comparing the child's height and weight against a growth chart, which ranks children in percentiles based on studies of height and weight distributions of large numbers of youngsters. A child who is in the fiftieth percentile for height, for example, is taller than half the children his age and shorter than the other half. If he ranks in the seventy-fifth percentile for both height and weight, he's probably big but not obese. But a child who is of average height and above-average weight is probably noticeably chubby.

Once you've determined your child is overweight, you're going to have to acquire some nutritional wisdom quickly. A child who is still growing can't go on the latest quirky diet and sweat it off at a spa.

"Adults can go on all sorts of crazy diets and their bodies adapt," says Kelly D. Brownell, Ph.D., codirector of the obesity research group at the University of Pennsylvania, in Philadelphia. "If you put a child on a radical diet, it can interfere with his growth. You have to be far more concerned about nutrition with a child."

Some children—those only moderately obese or overweight babies, for instance—do not need to lose weight at all.

For them, a maintenance diet is the best route. As they grow, height will take care of weight.

Parents should be aware from the onset that slimming down isn't easy for anyone, even children. But there are ways to make it less painful. Here's some of the latest advice from several of the country's leading obesity experts.

Catch It Early

How early? The experts agree: when junior begins to prematurely outgrow his swaddling clothes. Obesity is a problem that, like many killer diseases, has a high "cure" rate when caught and treated early: when children haven't acquired poor eating habits and parents still have some control over the food they eat.

It's also easier then. "A child under eight expects you to control him," says Warren Silberstein, M.D., a New York pediatrician and author of *Helping Your Child Grow Slim* (Simon & Schuster, 1982). "You control his bedtime, what he watches on TV, so there's no reason why food should be any different."

Parents tend to lose some influence over the eating habits of more-independent school-age youngsters who, at the same time they have candy money also have little motivation to lose weight. "A nine-year-old doesn't care what she looks like," says Dr. Sidbury, who has worked with overweight youngsters for 15 years. "Frequently you're batting your head against the wall until they become interested in the opposite sex."

But while prom gowns and communal gym showers sound like strong motivation, overweight teenagers have a dimmer dieting prognosis than younger children. By adolescence, poor eating habits may be already a decade old and overeating may have become an emotional outlet, serving as solace for dateless Saturdays or poor grades.

Sandy Lieberman is convinced that it's never too soon. Her son Timmy weighed only slightly over eight pounds at birth. But by the time he was three months old he was tipping the scales at 19 pounds, about the same weight as his older sister was at 15 months. "He had no cheeks and no neck," recalls Sandy, who also has three daughters. "When we brought him home the doctor told us we could start him on formula when he could take three ounces. He didn't start with three ounces. He had eight. He didn't start with one or two table-spoons of cereal, he had the whole bowl."

The actual slimming down procedure for the hefty infant can be fairly easy, as Sandy Lieberman discovered. On the advice of her pediatrician, she simply diluted Timmy's formula to keep his weight stable until he grew into it at a year and a half.

Some experts recommend substituting low-fat for whole milk and emphasizing low-fat meats, vegetables and fruit for overweight toddlers. "Usually controlling dietary fat is enough," says Alfred E. Slonim, M.D., director of the Obesity Clinic, a program for children and adolescents at North Shore University Medical Center in Manhasset, New York. "Fat has more than twice as many calories per gram as carbohydrates and protein."

Your pediatrician should be able to help you work out a plan for your child.

Parents will probably have to start a program of behavior modification as well—for themselves. The Timmys of the world are rare. ("A small number of these kids come out of the womb hungry as bears," says Dr. Sidbury.) More common are the infants whose mothers associate every wail with hunger or use the bottle as a pacifier.

Remember: Food Is Only Nourishment

Studies have shown that infants whose parents respond to their crying with food later tend to associate all kinds of feelings, from sadness to boredom, with hunger. Food should never be a substitute for love or attention, nor a reward for a good report card or clean room.

"You want Johnny to do it your way, so you give him a cookie," says Dr. Sidbury. "It's easy. You hand it out. The better thing is to use affection as a reward."

Dr. Sidbury also recommends that mothers, when they can, breastfeed infants. It helps a mother become more attuned to her child's hunger pattern. "When you breastfeed, the baby stops when he's had enough. With an eight-ounce bottle, the temptation is to jiggle it until he's had it all. Some mothers never learn how much their child really wants to eat."

Go on a Diet Yourself

Research shows that it's likely an overweight child has at least one overweight parent. If it's you, be your child's dieting buddy.

In his program, Dr. Sidbury found that when parents diet along with their youngster, "the chances of a child being successful go up."

Sometimes it works the other way around. When Jeri-Jean Thomas decided to shed 25 pounds—at age ten—her mother, Carol, was so impressed that she took off 50. Her father, Andy, dropped 65. "I started after she had reached her goal," says Mrs. Thomas. "I thought, if she can do it, there's no reason why I can't. She was my inspiration."

Give Positive Support

If the unmerciful teasing of other children doesn't help, your nagging isn't going to coerce your child into losing weight.

"Twenty-four hours of that is enough to drive someone to drink, much less eat," says Dee Matthews, coauthor of *The You Can Do It! Kids Diet* (Holt, Rinehart and Winston, 1985) and founder of Diet Encounter, a successful weight-control program for children in Palm Beach, Florida.

"If there's a food missing from the refrigerator, don't automatically accuse the fat child," says Mrs. Matthews, who was an overweight child herself. "Don't tell the whole neighborhood your child's lost weight. I tell the kids, it's your business, it's your body. Tell the child you're concerned, that you want to help. But don't ask, 'Did you drink all your water, did you eat your salad?' Let them do 99¾ percent of it. After all, they're going to reap all the rewards."

She encourages parents to allow the dieting child to take part in grocery shopping and meal preparation. It's often a break for the chief cook and bottle washer—whichever parent that may be—and a good lesson in responsibility for the child.

Keep Active

Most obesity studies have found that overweight people don't necessarily eat more than those of normal weight, but they are less active. Exercise has to go hand in hand with dieting.

But, like dieting, exercise programs for children have to be tailored to their special needs. "First of all, the words 'exercise program' connote something to people, usually pain and fatigue," says Dr. Brownell. "It's hard to get overweight people, even children, to exercise. It's not fun, it's boring and it hurts. But its not too hard to walk to the store or take the dog out or ride your bike. Studies have found that overweight people who get involved in a variety of lifestyle activities—like walking and bike riding—have better results."

Use Diet Tricks

What works for adults also works for children. Eating slowly, eating only at the table and quitting the "clean plate club" can help change bad habits.

"Give kids water between meals to fill them up," says Dr. Sidbury. "Don't feed them finger foods. It's too easy to overeat. Serve only foods you have to eat with a knife and a fork."

Behavior modification is the underpinning of the obesity research program at the University of Pennsylvania. Dr. Brownell has written a comprehensive workbook guide on what he calls the LEARN program for weight control. LEARN is an acronym for Lifestyle, Exercise, Attitudes, Relationships and Nutrition.

Filled with familiar cartoon figures such as Garfield and Cathy, the 215-page booklet can help a dieter with everything from keeping a food diary to learning the basic four food groups. Among its suggestions:

● Look for patterns in a food diary. When does the child snack? What are her favorite fattening foods? Does she overeat when she's feeling blue or bored or plopped in front of her favorite TV show? This can help identify eating triggers and high-risk situations that can be avoided.

● Walk. It's one exercise anyone can do. Many overweight children are embarrassed to exercise and may even find it too difficult. But a walking program can be adjusted for pace and ability.

● Find distractions. This is an easy one for children who tend to have good imaginations. When they're confronted by an "uncontrollable" craving for something to eat, encourage them to think about something else—buying a new, smaller-sized wardrobe, wearing a bathing suit on the beach. The craving usually passes.

● Develop alternative activities. It's tough to build a model airplane or ride a bike while eating a ham sandwich. Have the child make a list of all the activities that are incompatible with eating and tell him to consult the list when he gets the snacking urge. Make sure he lists only activities he would find enjoyable, because the alternatives have to be at least as satisfying as a candy bar would be.

For more information about Dr. Brownell's booklet, send a self-addressed stamped envelope to Dr. Kelly D. Brownell, Department of Psychiatry, University of Pennsylvania, 133 S. 36th St., Philadelphia, PA 19104.

Turn Off the Tube

Researchers at the New England Medical Center and Harvard School of Public Health, investigating the television-viewing habits of nearly 7,000 youngsters, discovered that the children who watched the most TV were more likely to be overweight, eat between-meal snacks and do poorly in school.

The scientists suggest that the prevalence of childhood obesity could be reduced and, in some cases, overweight could be prevented simply by reducing the amount of television children watch.

Fight the Food Myths

Number 1: Kids get fat on junk food.

Right? Wrong, says Dr. Silberstein. "Any child who is overweight is overeating all kinds of food. Parents make the mistake of thinking, if it's good for you it can't hurt. You have to cut down in balance. You have to understand that good food can cause you as big a weight problem as bad food."

Number 2: Kids won't eat foods that are good for them.

Wrong, says Dr. Sidbury. "No question, what a kid eats for a period of time he comes to prefer. This was seen when epileptics were still being given special diets. These were horrendous diets. Nauseating, actually. High in fat, with very little protein and carbohydrate. After two years, these kids no longer liked sweets. They wanted only high-fat foods."

If it's all they're served, the experts say, kids can grow to like salads and vegetables and shun anything sweeter than a fresh peach.

Health on the Home Front

Sweep Danger from Your Home

At first glance, it would appear that we are a careless lot. People are accidentally harming, disabling and killing themselves in their home sweet homes at record rates. Yet oddly enough, the victims aren't always negligent, unthinking simpletons who beg for accidents by leaving a bar of soap in the bathtub or tossing a loose rug across the stairs. Accidents are befalling careful, insightful people who have smoke detectors and sturdy banisters, and who think they've done as much as possible to make their homes safe.

Yet even the most safety-conscious homeowner might be unaware of the more obscure, almost invisible things around the house that aren't readily associated with accidents: aspects of everyday life that could cause serious problems if uncorrected. Sitting in an emergency room waiting to be stitched up is a bit late to realize there should have been a decal or a piece of tape at eye level on the sliding glass door you just walked through. And the split second before body meets floor is a poor time to discover there's no grab bar in the bathtub.

The Deceiving Comforts of Home

In the days of dinosaurs, our prehistoric ancestors lived relatively uncluttered lives and mainly had to be careful not to trip over a bone or sit on a spear when puttering around the cave. Today our domiciles are far more complicated, designed for privacy and equipped for our convenience and well-being. Unfortunately, the modern nuances make our lives more hazardous. Preventable incidents involving heating systems, bathing facilities, glass windows, doors, electricity, stairs and a variety of seemingly innocent items, such as automatic garage-door openers, are contributing to the rising accident statistics. The National Safety Council reports that an estimated 24.8 million people were injured in their homes in 1984. Accidental deaths in the home increased 2 percent over 1983, and disabling injuries were up 1 percent.

"Most people aren't knowledgeable about the accident possibilities around their houses," says Frank Vilardo, Dr.P.H., of the Indiana University Institute for Research and Public Safety, Bloomington. "People tend to think more about safety in the workplace because there are regulations that must be enforced and supervisors to make sure the standards are followed. When they get home they relax and feel safe in a comfortable environment where they don't feel they have to look for potential accidents."

While some adults apparently feel indestructible in their homes, many realize that their children and grandchildren are anything but superhuman. As a result, great strides have been made to make houses safe for youngsters, says Joseph Greensher, M.D., chairman of the American Academy of Pediatrics Committee on Accident and Poison Prevention.

"The change came about when we did away with the diseases that were claiming so many kids, and people realized that accidents were killing children," he says. "The concept of death has also changed. People used to believe that when a person died from an accident, it was an act of God and there was nothing that could be done. Now they realize they have more control over many aspects of everyday life and can do things to reduce the risks."

Avoiding the Falls

Falls are the leading cause of accidental deaths in the home, and head the list of accidents experienced by older adults, according to National Safety Council statistics. More than 80 percent of those killed by falls each year are over 65.

Most falls take place on stairs or steps, statistics show. Many trips and slips occur where there are only a few steps, such as on decks or walkways. Slight, abrupt elevation changes often go unnoticed, and the unexpected rise can throw a person off balance. In older houses, installing a slight ramp with a slip-resistant surface would remove the accident potential.

Stairs inside the house are safer if covered with nonskid material, such as rubber mats or treads. If stairs are carpeted, shag and deep-pile types reduce the width of each step and could make for unsure footing. Carpets and rugs with rich patterns can mask the edge of the steps and make it hard to tell where one ends and another begins.

"Handrails are essential where there are more than three steps, and they should be rounded for the best possible grip," says Ravi Waldon, director of the American Institute of Architects housing program, Washington, D.C. It's also a good idea to install a handrail about two feet above the steps for children.

Banisters can be dangerous for young children. Since an inquisitive child will often try to stick his head through a railing, openings should be no more than five inches. A similar hazard occurs when a child gets his head caught beneath the bottom rail of a banister that stops a few inches from the floor. One youngster was severely injured when he slid on a marble floor in an East Coast concert hall and jammed his head between the floor and rail. The accident pointed to a safety hazard that had gone unnoticed and codes were modified to alert builders to the potential problem.

Another treacherous area is the bathroom, where most accidents occur when entering or leaving the tub, or while changing positions. The U.S. Department of Commerce estimates that bathtub and shower accidents cost an estimated $78.5 million annually in medical bills and lost work time.

Tubs should have nonslip or textured bottoms or a bath mat. Firm, unbreakable grab bars should be installed in the bathing area. Don't make the mistake of thinking that a towel rack or soap dish screwed into the wall will stop a fall.

The bathroom floor should also have a nonskid surface, or at least rugs to soak up the inevitable puddles.

To lessen the impact of a fall, add-on edges made of resilient material can be bought or designed for tubs, and a soft seat and cover can be installed on toilets. When designing a house, recessing the soap dish, faucet and controls could reduce the severity of a fall.

Portals to Accidents

Doors and windows that separate the outside from the inside are another source of potential accidents. Garage doors are especially hazardous to both young and old, and even safety experts aren't immune to accidents in the garage, as Dr. Vilardo learned.

"I had thought about calling a repairman to fix a spring on my garage door, but then decided I'd save the money and do it myself," he says. "It seemed simple enough, but when I released the spring, there was a lot of tension and it caught my hand between the door and spring.

"This is a typical approach to a problem around the house. People usually don't have the tools or knowledge to fix something, but they cheat and get away with it a few times. They keep on cheating until they get careless and have an accident. I saved $30 in repair bills but lost $500 in medical expenses and aggravation."

Electric garage-door openers can also be hazardous, especially to children. Two Minnesota children were killed in separate incidents when they were caught beneath closing doors. While newer models stop or reverse the door when an object is encountered, older models may not have the safety feature, which means the controls should be out of reach of young hands or locked inside the car.

If you open your garage door by hand it's the type with several folding sections, handles should be attached to each section so fingers won't be mashed while closing the door.

Elsewhere in the house, double-action swinging doors should have padding at the doorjamb to minimize injury to pinched fingers. Thresholds on inside doors can cause stumbles, and should be removed unless needed to maintain a level walking surface.

Window walls or sliding glass doors are aesthetically pleasing, but should consist of safety glass, which may be missing in older homes. To keep a child from plunging through the glass, a sill or other guard, such as a planter, decorative railing or furniture, should stretch across the glass about 12 inches above floor level.

Screens can keep bugs out but don't guarantee that children will stay in, so don't arrange furniture in such a way that youngsters can stand in windows. Metal locks can be installed to limit the height a window can be opened. To prevent fingers from being mashed, second stops can be installed.

A Shockingly Current Problem

You turn on electricity with the flip of a switch, forgetting how easily it can turn you on, usually when there's water around.

Electrical hazards are an unending source of danger in twentieth-century bathrooms, which are stocked with hair dryers, razors, curlers, radios, hot lather dispensers and even televisions and tape players. Electrocutions can occur when people in the tub or still wet come in contact with a switch or appliance. The safest preventives are to ensure that electrical apparatuses can't reach the tub, sink, toilet or shower, and that the devices are unplugged when not in use.

Since it's probably impossible to remove all electrical items from the bathroom, ground fault circuit interrupters should be wired into circuits at panel boxes or used to replace ordinary outlets. A GFCI prevents shock by monitoring circuits and shutting off power if leakage to another ground, or source, is detected. Many local building codes now require GFCIs for outdoor receptacles, bathrooms, garages and other applications. Older houses are rarely equipped with GFCIs, and an electrician should be contacted about installation. In newer houses, check outlets or the circuit-breaker box for little red test buttons that pop out when there's a problem with the circuit.

In bathrooms in many older homes, the light over the sink

is turned on by yanking a chain. If a short develops, touching the chain and the metal faucet can put a person in the middle of an electrical circuit, since the body will lead the charge to the nearest ground—the faucet. To prevent a shock, an insulating link should be installed near the socket, or the chain should be replaced with some type of nonconductive material, such as cord.

Some Like It Hot

The household heating system usually only comes to mind when temperatures drop, but it should be checked before each winter. Homeowners should know where fuel cutoffs are in case of emergency, and fuel lines shouldn't extend into areas where the lines can be easily damaged.

Any stationary fuel-consuming heating device should be vented to the outside, and the vent system should be checked annually for leaks. Older units may require more frequent inspections. The National Safety Council reports that gas heating devices account for 290 of the estimated 340 carbon-monoxide poisoning deaths each year. In spaces that are well insulated, fairly airtight and heated by nonvented units, fresh air should be supplied by opening a window at least one-half inch.

If a fireplace is used for either heat or aesthetics, the hearth should extend at least 21 to 24 inches into the room to prevent sparks from igniting the rug or nearby materials. Flame-retardant pads can be added if necessary. Outside, the chimney should be in good repair. For a good draft, most codes require that the chimney be at least two feet taller than any point on the roof that is ten feet or less away horizontally; otherwise, smoke may be sucked into the house. Rather than hiring a brick mason, prefabricated metal chimney extensions can be purchased.

It may be impossible to guarantee a home free of potential accidents since there will always be things to look out for. With your house in mind, consider the following:

● Showers should be equipped with temperature-regulating valves to keep the water in the bath a constant temperature even when the kitchen faucet is turned on to wash potatoes, for example. Otherwise scalds can occur when the chilly bather turns up the hot water just before the potato washer finishes downstairs.

● Cabinet drawers should have catches so they won't pull all the way out and drop on toes.

● Clothes hooks on the back of bathroom and bedroom doors should be above eye level.

● Rounded edges on cabinets and furniture are more difficult for the carpenter, "but they are safer," says Jim Presswood, occupational safety and fire-protection officer, University of Texas Health Science Center, Dallas. "You'll get bruised if you hit a rounded edge, but chances are you won't be disabled or killed."

"Accident prevention around the home requires a constant effort because there are so many hidden hazards," says Dr. Vilardo. "There's not the same degree of concern for home safety as there is for highway safety, so it's up to the individual homeowner to be aware that there are things that can be done to make a house safer."

How to Avoid Food Poisoning

If you think food poisoning is a thing of the past, consider this: In March and April, 1985, more than 17,000 people in five midwestern states became sick with salmonellosis. They suffered the abdominal pain, nausea, diarrhea, vomiting and fever that infection with *salmonella* bacteria causes. At least two deaths were directly attributed to the bacteria. The outbreak, the nation's largest, was traced to contaminated milk.

There was no way those people could have known the danger: The bacteria was colorless, odorless and tasteless. And although an outbreak of that magnitude is unusual, food poisoning itself is common.

"We estimate that in 1984 there were more than 4 million

cases of salmonellosis," says Patricia Griffin, M.D., an epidemiologist at the Centers for Disease Control, located in Atlanta. "One study estimated that the total cost of caring for patients with salmonella poisoning is $1 billion a year."

No need to lock yourself in a sterile environment, though. Most food poisoning is the result of human error, and you can often protect yourself if you know the basics of food sanitation.

Cast of Characters

There are over 1,800 strains of *salmonella,* and most of them can cause food poisoning. But there are other culprits, too. *Staphylococcus aureus, Clostridium botulinum* and *Clostridium perfringens* are three of the most well-known.

There are two ways they can cause trouble. True food poisoning is caused by eating food containing poison or toxin produced by bacteria growing in the food. Botulism and staphylococcal food poisoning are this type. The second type, a food-borne infection, is caused by eating food containing organisms that grow (with bacteria, that means multiply) in the body. Salmonellosis is an example of this type. Although this may sound complicated, keeping the organisms in check is easy.

And keeping them in check is the goal. The bacteria that cause most food poisonings are everywhere, including in our food. So rather than trying to get rid of them (an impossible task), prevention of poisoning is a matter of stopping their growth or killing them at the proper time.

According to Dr. Griffin, there are five common mistakes that can cause food-borne disease. Avoid them and you can keep your food safe.

1. *Improper holding temperature* is responsible for most reported cases of food poisoning. "Many illnesses come from church picnics, where the food is prepared earlier, taken out and held for hours," says Tom Schwarz, assistant director for program development in the retail-food-protection branch of the Food and Drug Administration.

Most bacteria are killed by temperatures above 165°F. They are prevented from growing at temperatures above 150° or below 40°F. But in between, they grow very quickly (the warmer, the quicker). Keep food at those in-between temperatures and you're looking for trouble, especially if you hold it for more than two hours.

"There is one very simple rule," says Edmund A. Zottola, Ph.D., professor of food microbiology in the department of food science and nutrition at the University of Minnesota in St. Paul. "Either keep it hot or keep it cold."

It's unwise, for example, to let a hot dish cool on the counter before putting it in the refrigerator. As it cools gradually, it spends a lot of time in the optimum growing temperature range for bacteria. "The aim is to cool food to 40° within four hours," says Schwarz. The food will cool off much quicker in the refrigerator.

But you have to use common sense, too. "If you put a five-gallon stew pot in the refrigerator, it might warm everything up, particularly if you have a small, apartment-size refrigerator," says Dr. Zottola. "And it won't cook quickly enough. If you've made a large pot of chili, put it in smaller containers so it cools faster."

Take care to keep raw foods refrigerated, too. If a piece of meat is contaminated with *staphylococcus* (there's no way to know what's in there), and it sits at room temperature for hours, the meat may be loaded with toxin by the time you cook it. And the toxin is not destroyed by heating.

Think far enough ahead to thaw foods in the refrigerator. If you must leave them out, thaw them in sealed packages under cold water. And try to have the refrigerator door open as briefly and infrequently as possible, to make sure it stays at 40°F.

2. *Inadequately cooked food* is also a danger. Raw chicken, for example, is highly contaminated with *salmonella* and *campylobacter.* One study by researchers at Iowa State University found *salmonella* in 40.7 percent of packaged cutup chickens.

You can avoid problems by throughly cooking meat, poultry and seafood. As a general rule, cooking those foods to an internal temperature of 165°F should kill any freeloading bacteria. That goes for leftovers as well. They should be reheated to 165°F, not just warmed up.

Tasting foods while they're cooking is also hazardous. So-called Jewish Mothers' Disease was a problem when women used to make their own gefilte fish. It came from tasting fish before it was thoroughly cooked. It was caused by a parasite in the raw fish.

3. *Poor personal hygiene* is another cause of food poisoning. That's why hand washing is so important. "It's particularly important after going to the bathroom," says Schwarz, "because the worst organisms for food-borne illness are fecally transmitted."

The code for institutional food services and restaurants says that you shouldn't smoke while handling food. "The reason has nothing to do with cigarettes," says Schwarz. "It has to do with putting your hand in your mouth. When you smoke, you touch the end of the cigarette, you get saliva on your fingers and you transmit it to the food. For the same reason, the code requires hand washing after smoking, eating and drinking." Tasting food can transmit germs too. To be safe, use a clean spoon each time you taste.

"If you're sick, you probably shouldn't be handling food," cautions Dr. Zottola. "The same is true if you have an infected cut, skin irritation, boils or acne."

4. *Contaminated equipment* has been traced to many outbreaks of food-borne disease. It may be obvious that you should use clean utensils when preparing food. But not knowing just what constitutes "clean" has caused many an upset stomach.

Here's a common scenario: You cut up a raw chicken on a wooden cutting board. Then you cut up vegetables for a salad, using the same knife and cutting board. Did you spot your three mistakes?

Raw chicken frequently harbors bacteria. When you cut it up, bacteria gets on your hands and on the knife, and soak into the porous cutting board. If you then use your hands, the knife and the cutting board to prepare a salad, the bacteria are transmitted to the vegetables, which will not be cooked.

After handling raw meat or poultry, always scrub your hands, utensils and cutting board thoroughly with soap and hot water to prevent cross-contamination. Adding a little chlorine bleach to the rinse helps. Having two cutting boards, one for meat and one for vegetables, can help avoid problems, too. Just make sure the one used for meat gets sanitized. One of the best methods for sanitizing your implements is running them through the dishwasher.

5. *Food from an unsafe source* should be avoided if you don't want to risk food poisoning. "Eating raw meat or seafood is not completely safe," says Dr. Griffin. "You're taking a risk. There could be bacteria in them. We strongly advise against drinking raw milk, too. Despite its reputation as a healthy food, raw milk has been the cause of quite a number of outbreaks of food-borne disease, because it can carry bacteria. Pasteurization is the best thing that ever happened to milk."

Dirty or cracked eggs also should not be used. The dirt might be chicken manure, teeming with bacteria. But mayonnaise, despite all the bad press, is seldom a cause of food poisoning. It is too acid for bacteria to grow in easily. It's not until it's diluted with other foods, such as eggs, tuna or macaroni, that it becomes a medium for bacterial growth. Acidic and sugary foods generally do not support the growth of bacteria, although they may eventually grow mold (see "Breaking the Mold," page 263).

Buying Trouble

You can be very careful to handle food properly in your home, but how can you tell if the food you buy at the market is safe? You can't, for the most part. "You have to rely on the quality control of the manufacturers," says Schwarz. Of course, they have a lot of incentive. One outbreak traced to a manufacturer's food can mean the end of his business.

Surprisingly, expiration dates are of little help. "The dates are set by the manufacturers and reflect changes in quality," says Schwarz. "On that date, for example, a package of cheese is not necessarily hazardous or unfit. It's just that the quality goes down." Still, the less time a quart of milk has been hanging around, the better.

Avoid foods that have an off odor or color. Put perishables in your shopping basket just before going to the checkout and refrigerate them promptly. Use meats, poultry and seafood as soon as possible.

You're just as vulnerable to food poisoning when you eat out, because restaurants are associated with about half of all outbreaks of food-borne disease. "You put an awful lot of faith in people when you eat in a restaurant," says Dr. Zottola. "It's like driving a car. You know *you're* going to do it right but you worry about the other guy." With good reason. It's not required that restaurant personnel have training in proper food-handling procedures.

And it's hard to judge a restaurant without seeing what goes on in the kitchen. But there are some things you can look for. "You can see if the restaurant is clean generally," says Schwarz. "Is there spilled food that looks like it's been sitting there for hours?

"I check that the food is cooked well, and that hot foods are hot and cold foods are cold. I won't eat warm tuna salad—it hasn't been kept in the refrigerator. And I send back soups or stews that are only lukewarm."

Be wary of foods that take a lot of handling in their preparation, such as potato salad or stew, and of the foods most likely to harbor bacteria. "We use the term 'potentially hazardous food' to describe a food that supports the rapid and progressive growth of pathogenic and toxigenic organisms," says Schwarz. "They include most meat, poultry, seafood, fish and milk products, and cooked vegetables."

If you have vomiting or diarrhea and you think you have contracted food poisoning from dining out or from a commercially canned or processed food, call your local health department. They may be able to save others from your fate. The problem is, it's hard to tell if you've got food poisoning or a stomach virus, because the symptoms can be so similar.

It may take a couple of days for *salmonella* to make you sick with diarrhea, because it takes time for the bacteria to grow in your intestinal tract. If you're severely ill for a few days, call your doctor, because severe cases can be dangerous. If you've eaten *staphylococcus* toxin, you'll get sick within one to six hours, and should be over it in a day or two, as soon as the vomiting and diarrhea rid your body of the toxin.

Turkey Trots

Do you like to celebrate holidays by making a big turkey dinner? You probably try to prepare as much as possible ahead of time. That's okay, with one exception: stuffing the turkey. Do that ahead of time and your celebration could be no holiday.

Here's why. Raw turkey harbors *salmonella* bacteria. If you pack a bird tightly with warm stuffing, the bacteria will have all night to multiply, even though it's refrigerated. The cold just can't penetrate to the center of the turkey fast enough.

Same problem with cooking the turkey. Be sure that the center reaches 165°F, the temperature necessary to kill *salmonella*. And if the turkey was contaminated with *staphylococcus* bacteria, even thorough cooking couldn't save you—the toxin isn't destroyed by heat.

Breaking the Mold

Molds grow in the refrigerator because they can tolerate the low temperature. But they're unwelcome guests. They can hasten food spoilage and cause allergic and respiratory problems. And under the right conditions, some molds can produce mycotoxins, or poisons.

What should you do if the fuzzies pay a visit to your refrigerator? Here are some recommendations from the U.S. Department of Agriculture:

Don't sniff the moldy item—molds can cause respiratory problems. If the food is heavily covered with mold, wrap it gently and discard it immediately. Clean the refrigerator where the food was sitting and examine nearby items.

If the food has only a tiny spot of mold, proceed as follows:

● In hard-block cheeses, cut off at least an inch around and below the mold spot. Keep your knife out of the mold. Rewrap in fresh wrap. The same procedure can be followed for hard salami and smoked turkey.

● In jams and jellies, a tiny spot of mold can be scooped out. With a second, clean spoon, scoop out more jam around the spot. If the rest looks and smells normal, it's okay. If it tastes fermented, throw it out.

● In firm vegetables, such as cabbage and carrots, you can cut away small spots of mold from the surface. But you should discard soft vegetables, such as tomatoes, cucumbers and lettuce, if they show mold growth.

● Discard moldy soft cheese, cottage cheese, cream, sour cream, yogurt, individual cheese slices, bacon, hot dogs, sliced lunch meats, meat pies, opened canned ham, baked chicken, bread, cake, buns, pastry, corn, nuts, flour, whole grains, rice, dried peas and beans, and peanut butter.

Botulism: Rare but Deadly

Botulism is a food-borne disease caused by *Clostridium botulinum*, bacteria that produce a deadly toxin, or poison, when they grow in food. About 30 percent of the people who become sick with botulism die. Scientists estimate that one cupful of this toxin could kill all the people on earth.

Luckily, botulism is rare. There are only 10 to 15 cases each year in the United States. Although a few are traced to commercially canned or processed foods, about 75 percent of the cases are caused by improperly home-canned foods.

Never eat or even taste food from a swollen can or jar, or food that is foamy, moldy or has a bad odor from a can or jar. Dispose of the food in such a way that there is no chance it will be eaten by humans or animals.

Always boil home-canned vegetables and never taste them before cooking them. The toxin that causes botulism is destroyed by heat. Bringing the food to a boil and holding it there for a few minutes inactivates the toxin.

If you intend to do home canning, be sure you are using the proper techniques. Your local Agricultural Extension Service may publish a booklet on home canning. If not, they can refer you to a reliable source.

For more information on preventing food-borne diseases you can write the Meat and Poultry Hotline, USDA Food Safety and Inspection Service, Room 1163 South, Washington, DC 20250, or call 800-535-4555 (in the Washington, DC, area, call 447-3333). Or contact your local Agricultural Extension Service.

Do You Need a Band-Aid ... or an Ambulance?

"I've been seeing patients, thousands of them, for 15 years," says Bruce Janiak, M.D., director of the emergency center at Toledo Hospital, in Toledo, Ohio. "And, sure, I get frustrated when somebody comes in with a minor problem. But it is reassuring to the patient to find out that somebody says you're not dying and you don't have a major problem."

Dr. Janiak, current president of the American College of Emergency Physicians, lives by this credo: If a patient feels that a medical problem is an emergency, then it should be treated as such.

Some critics suspect such a sentiment encourages patients to visit hospital emergency departments when they don't really need emergency treatment. But Dr. Janiak doesn't think so.

"This view is in contrast to those people who are constantly telling us there are patients who abuse the emergency department," says Dr. Janiak. "We recognize that that happens, but it isn't as often as people say. And the overall impact on the public appears to be positive. There are many disease processes that are caught in time. Waiting until they're worse, until they become a terrible emergency, doesn't save anybody anything."

Emergencies Not Always Apparent

When nearsighted Uncle Ned has a mishap with the chain saw, the sudden and unexpected loss of his fingers or toes is, without question, a bona-fide emergency. But it isn't always easy for a lay-person to tell the difference between trivial trauma and and a matter of life and death.

Take, for example, the true story of a man who went to an emergency department complaining of a toothache. The admitting nurse took the man's pulse and realized his heartbeat was irregular. A few tests later came the diagnosis: myocardial infarction—a heart attack.

Pain from heart attack can "radiate" to the arms and jaw. In this instance, aside from the pain in his jaw, the man felt no discomfort.

"The body responds in different ways for different people," explains Dr. Janiak. "Different people have different pain thresholds. You cut off a leg and some people don't even whimper. You can have a fly land on other people and they faint from the pain."

Often, people suspect they might need prompt medical attention, but they aren't sure.

"We can't make everybody in the world a doctor," says Dr.

Janiak. "So you've got to have someplace where you can go to seek advice."

In a nationwide study, conducted jointly by the American Medical Association and the American College of Emergency Physicians, 45 percent of all people surveyed said they would not seek emergency medical assistance for shortness of breath. Seventy percent said they did not think they needed emergency aid for dizziness. Yet both these symptoms *could* be—though certainly not in all cases—early warning signs of heart attack or other serious illness.

Even the doctor sometimes can't tell what's wrong with you until he or she examines you and orders up a few diagnostic tests, says Dr. Janiak. And if the doctor can't tell what's wrong at first sight, it's even more unlikely that you can. Even so, it is possible for a health-care consumer to make an informed decision to seek emergency medical assistance.

Most people recognize severe bleeding or broken bones as genuine emergencies, says Dr. Janiak. The problem is recognizing less obvious symptoms as potentially serious health problems in need of immediate care. According to the American College of Emergency Physicians, there are seven warning signs of potential medical emergencies:

● Pain or pressure in your chest or upper abdomen
● Vomiting, when it is severe or continuous
● Fainting
● Dizziness, a sudden feeling of weakness or a severe change in vision
● Shortness of breath, or trouble breathing
● Severe pain anywhere in your body
● Homicidal or suicidal feelings.

Some of these warning signs may be as painfully obvious as they are painful. Others are less so. The key to knowing when to go for emergency help is suddenness.

"If the patient is having chest pains that scare him, he ought to come right in to the emergency department," says Dr. Janiak. "In general, the more sudden the change, the more reason to come right in."

If you have what appears to be a relatively minor problem,

but you aren't sure, Dr. Janiak believes it is reasonable to call your family doctor. Your doctor can tell you whether your problem deserves prompt attention in an emergency setting or whether it can wait for a routine office visit.

"If you can't contact your doctor," he adds, "a lot of emergency departments are willing to discuss it with you on the phone. I'm happy to tell people they don't need to come in. We're busy enough."

You Do Have Rights

You might be perplexed by the reception you get when you wander into the local emergency department gingerly cradling a bruised, swollen forearm or holding a crumpled handkerchief over a bleeding finger. After all, the sign on the door reads, in big red letters, EMERGENCY, right?

So why isn't everybody jumping up and down trying to help you?

It isn't that simple. What looks like an emergency to you might not be an emergency in the eyes of the staff nurse or doctor.

More than 77 million Americans make the trip to emergency departments every year—and the numbers are increasing at the rate of about 10 percent annually. ED visits have increased by 600 percent since World War II.

Clearly, in the chaos of the emergency department, many patients feel they have been slighted or overlooked. But patients *do* have rights, even in the midst of chaos.

"I think the public does have a right to expect reasonably fast evaluation of their problems," says Dr. Janiak. "They *don't* have a right to expect any treatment for it. The reason it has to be that way is, the treatment you might demand when you come in could be a shot of morphine because you think that's neat. But you don't have a right to that. You have a right to have me take a look at you and decide what I think you need and, together, we can discuss that."

Emergencies are, by definition, sudden and unexpected. It makes sense to decide what you're going to do *before* you drop the bowling ball on your foot or have an uncomfortably close encounter with Aunt Gert's attack dog.

The place to start is with your family doctor.

To begin with, is your doctor available to answer your medical questions 24 hours a day? If so, he or she could save you an unnecessary trip to the hospital.

"A lot of doctors are available 24 hours," says James D. Leitzell, M.D., who worked in Seattle-area emergency departments for eight years. "My recommendation to patients is that they establish a relationship with a doctor they trust who does make himself available. I think a person who is willing to call himself a doctor should accept the responsibility of being available for odd-hour calls. Many doctors do this. If you find yourself hooked up with a doctor who takes off on the weekends and isn't available when you need him, then you should consider finding somebody else."

The next step is to find out what hospital emergency department your doctor would recommend in the event you need one.

"I recognize the answer you're going to get is to go to the hospital that your doctor patronizes," says ACEP's Dr. Janiak. "That's not so bad because there is a continuity of record keeping. If a patient needs to be admitted, it saves transporting to another hospital. In an emergency, those conveniences are fairly important. The emergency department also should be close to where the patient lives. Then, finally, the choice should be based on the quality of the emergency department itself."

On the last point, again, Dr. Janiak believes the patient probably will have to trust the judgment of his or her physician.

In an emergency, every second counts. You can save time by posting your local emergency numbers alongside your telephone. It also helps either to have training in basic first aid or to keep written first-aid tips handy. If someone in your family has a heart problem, says Dr. Janiak, other members ought to be trained in cardiopulmonary resuscitation.

Finally, it helps to know a little bit about your local emergency services and how and when to use them.

Many areas of the country now are served by ambulance crews trained to handle most emergencies. Emergency medical technicians (EMTs) and paramedics—EMTs with advanced life-support training—represent a fundamental change in the way communities cope with emergencies.

In the past, the fellow who drove the ambulance might also have been the person at the wheel of the undertaker's hearse. EMTs are trained to assess your condition and begin appropriate care before and during the ride to the hospital. Frequently, the ambulances are equipped with radios so they can notify the hospital they're coming and provide detailed information about the patient's condition.

In other words, the ambulance is more than a taxi service, although it's often perceived as just that.

The question, then, is when to call the ambulance.

"If you have chest pain or trouble breathing, providing your own transportation is risky," says Dr. Janiak. "If you have a potentially serious injury—for example, you're riding your bike and get hit by a car—your own transportation is risky."

Even if you aren't the one who needs the doctor, it might be unwise for you to drive.

"The problem is, if the patient deteriorates on the way, the driver gets very anxious. Then he starts speeding. The patient collapses and the driver gets so hysterical that he could kill them both, not to mention some other people."

Under certain conditions, a patient should not be moved by anyone but trained ambulance personnel. If you suspect a person has broken his neck, back, thigh or pelvis, has broken several bones or has head injuries, you should not attempt to move the victim. Wait for trained emergency personnel.

For a free emergency-first-aid pamphlet, prepared by the American College of Emergency Physicians, write to: Communications Department, McNeil Consumer Products Co., Camp Hill Rd., Fort Washington, PA 19034.

Choosing and Using an Emergency Department

All emergency departments are not the same.

Here are six questions to ask, both before you need emergency medical care and when you need it, with answers from June Thompson, R.N., an assistant professor at the University of Texas Health Science Center at Houston School of Nursing.

Before You Need Emergency Care ●

1. Are the doctors and nurses certified in emergency care?

"I would certainly want to know what kind of physician coverage the facility has," says Thompson. "There is now a specialty in medicine called emergency medicine. There are now board-certified emergency physicians. There is also a certification program for emergency nursing.

"If I was picking a hospital I would want to know that the people I'm going to see are specialists in their area."

To find out if emergency medical personnel are certified, call your local hospitals and ask.

2. What kind of emergency department is it?

Hospital emergency departments now are classified according to the kind of treatment provided. For example, some emergency departments are full-fledged trauma centers, meaning doctors and nurses trained to handle serious injuries and medical emergencies are in the hospital, round the clock, with surgical facilities immediately available.

Other emergency departments may be staffed by family physicians, interns or doctors who are, essentially, moonlighting. Additionally, in some emergency departments, physicians are on call. They have to be summoned from somewhere else in the hospital or from home.

"I would want to know if the hospital has physicians in the hospital 24 hours a day, or does the nurse have to pick up the phone and call somebody," says Thompson. Of course, she adds, in some small communities served by only one hospital, there may be little choice.

"If I have a child, I want to know what kind of pediatricians they have available," Thompson says.

"I would go to one hospital, perhaps, if I were sick and to another hospital if I were injured, and that's where the trauma-center categorization comes in."

Some emergency departments may hang up a sign that says the facility is a trauma center. That doesn't mean it is certified as such. Only two national organizations can designate an emergency department as a trauma center, says Thompson: the Joint Commission on the Accreditation of

Hospitals and the American College of Surgeons. Again, call your local hospital to find out.

3. You've summoned an ambulance. Can you tell the driver to take you to the hospital of your own choosing?

It's possible, but in general, says Thompson, trust your local municipal or volunteer ambulance service to know what's best. "They know which hospitals to go to for trauma, for example, and they know which hospital to go to for pediatrics," Thompson says. "I think if you've got a good emergency-medical-services team in your community, I would trust that team." You *do* have the right to refuse ambulance transportation.

Once You Get There ●

4. Does a nurse or doctor examine me within five minutes after I arrive?

If the answer is yes, says Thompson, your local emergency department is performing up to accepted standards. A qualified emergency nurse ought to ask you what's wrong, take your vital signs—pulse, blood pressure and respiration—and determine your medical history. He or she may perform a preliminary examination or order diagnostic tests.

5. Are patients treated in the order of their arrival?

Usually not, if your local hospital uses what is called a triage system. *Triage* is a French word. Roughly translated, it means, "to sort."

In a triage system, says Thompson, patients with the most serious or potentially life- or limb-threatening problems are treated first. Those who suffer less serious problems are seen next. The least serious are seen last.

6. Am I asked for my insurance cards before a nurse or doctor takes my pulse and blood pressure and asks about my medical history?

Many of us have had the experience of entering the emergency department with what we think is a bona-fide emergency and being directed to a receptionist instead of to a doctor. That shouldn't happen. "If they do that," says Thompson, "I do not believe they have a functioning triage system."

Six Common Emergencies
and How to Recognize Them

Hospital emergency-department files are filled with cases of heartburn that turned out to be heart *attack*. And there are other pains that may seem minor but could be the signs of a serious medical emergency.

To help you recognize these potential emergencies, we've put together a list of six common complaints, with the cooperation of Richard Braen, M.D., secretary-treasurer of the American College of Emergency Physicians and director of the emergency department at Newton–Wellesley Hospital in Newton, Massachusetts.

Chest Pain ● It can be caused by many things, and it doesn't necessarily mean you're having a heart attack.

"You should be particularly concerned if the pain is a gripping type of chest pain underneath the breastbone that goes into the left arm, the neck and sometimes into the back," Dr. Braen says. "The type of pain is commonly crushing, squeezing. A lot of people describe it as 'somebody sitting on my chest.' It increases with time."

Heart-attack pain usually lasts longer than 20 minutes and can last one or more hours, he adds.

If the chest pain is caused by heart attack, you may suffer from nausea, vomiting, profuse sweating, shortness of breath and, occasionally, upper abdominal pain or fainting.

These could be the early signs of heart attack and should be taken seriously. If you observe these symptoms in yourself or someone else, you should seek emergency aid without delay. Don't try to get to the hospital by yourself, Dr. Braen advises. Rather, call your local ambulance service.

Abdominal Pain ● Here again, the possibilities are numerous, since the abdomen contains a number of vital organs. "One of the causes at the top of the list is acute appendicitis," says Dr. Braen.

"Generally, most people who have it are in their teens through thirties, but it can literally occur at any time in life.

"It often comes on gradually. Most people have a feeling of mild abdominal tenderness that gets increasingly severe, generally around the belly button, very frequently associated with loss of appetite. It may localize to the right lower side of the abdomen. If you have vomiting with it, generally, the vomiting comes *after* the abdominal pain. If vomiting comes first, we have less suspicion that it's appendicitis, even though it can exist.

"It can be associated with a low-grade fever and, less commonly, diarrhea."

If you suspect appendicitis, call your doctor and ask his opinion first, says Dr. Braen. Then, if you have to go to the hospital, he adds, you probably can be driven by private car.

One not of caution: If you suffer all the previously described symptoms and the pain is suddenly relieved, the appendix may have burst. This is a serious medical problem that requires immediate attention.

Diarrhea and Vomiting ● Prolonged diarrhea and vomiting can cause significant loss of body fluids, triggering shock.

Most people who have diarrhea or vomiting don't need to go to the emergency department, says Dr. Braen. However, if you can't keep liquids down, if you aren't urinating, have severe dizziness when you sit up or increased pulse, you ought to see a doctor.

Headache ● Everybody gets headaches. Most of them are associated with stress or fatigue. But, in general, says Dr. Braen, physicians are concerned about headaches that often are described by the patient as "the worst headache of my life."

Associated with fever or neck stiffness, the pain from this headache could be the outward sign of a burst blood vessel in the brain or meningitis. Severe headaches also could be the warning signals of dangerously high blood pressure, tumors and other problems.

"In most cases, one could contact the private doctor first," Dr. Braen says. "If that's unsuccessful and the headache is worse despite taking aspirin, the person definitely should come to the emergency department to be diagnosed."

Poisoning ● All sorts of things cause poisoning—for example, common household cleaners, detergents, drain openers, petroleum products and drugs. Dr. Braen strongly recommends you keep the number of your local poison information center handy and, when necessary, call that number first. It's often in the front of the telephone book.

It's also wise, if you have children, to keep a bottle of syrup of ipecac handy. Ipecac causes vomiting. However, Dr. Braen warns, *do not* try to induce vomiting until you've first consulted with a poison information center, emergency department or your private physician.

Fever in Children ● It's very common, as parents know. If the fever doesn't go down after you've administered aspirin or acetaminophen and sponged down the child, and it lasts more than a few hours, call your pediatrician, Dr. Braen advises.

More terrifying is when a child suddenly has a seizure caused by high fever.

"Any child who has had a seizure associated with a fever should be evaluated as soon as possible," says Dr. Braen, either by the pediatrician or in the emergency department.

Your Cheapest Life Insurance Policy

Maybe ten-year-old Elizabeth said it best when she said to her father, "But, Dad, you can't be healthy if you're dead."

Dad, in a hurry to get home before dark so he could go for a jog, had neglected to buckle his seat belt—a mistake a whopping *three-quarters* of the U.S. population make every day. In the words of health researcher Suzanne Irvine, "It just doesn't make sense."

And indeed it doesn't. Irvine was project manager of a recent nationwide survey (done by Louis Harris and Associates for *Prevention*), which found that while we're knuckling down in nearly all other aspects of health, we're still strangely remiss at buckling up.

"Eighty-seven percent of us are making efforts to cut down on alcohol or cut it out altogether; 72 percent of us are not smoking; 85 percent are keeping an eye on blood pressure; and better than half of us are making specific efforts to improve our diets," according to Irvine.

But how many of us are taking a few seconds a day buckling up to reduce by 50 percent our chances of being killed in a car accident?

"Only about one-quarter." Irvine says. "More of us—33 percent—are taking the time to exercise on a regular basis than to buckle up."

So the big question, of course, is *why.* Could it be that seat belts aren't effective, and the average driver knows something that the police and safety officials don't?

Very unlikely. Out of a total of 65 health-protecting behaviors considered in the *Prevention* survey—all of which were scrutinized by a team of leading doctors and health experts around the country—wearing seat belts ranked *fourth* in terms of overall importance for safeguarding health. Only "not smoking," "avoiding dependency on drugs" and "not smoking in bed" nudged out seat belts. The National Highway Traffic Safety Administration estimates that 17,000 lives could be saved every year if we'd all buckle up. And that 4 million injuries could be minimized dramatically. Seat belts—if worn—can work. All we've got to do is get into the habit of using them.

Indeed, studies suggest that the biggest reason more of us aren't buckling up is simply that we haven't been trained to. Already our children (e.g., Elizabeth) are better at buckling up than we are because the wisdom of seat belts is being taught in the schools. For most drivers of today, however (many of whom were on the road long before seat belts came into existence), the idea of strapping oneself in is quite alien. Their idea of operating an automobile, unfortunately, is simply to get in and get going.

The no-seat-belt habit is one that can be broken, however. All it takes is concentrated effort to make it a specific point to buckle up. As one recent seat-belt convert told us, " I now feel a little naked if I'm *not* buckled up. I've gotten attached to the feeling of security my seat belt gives me."

But force of habit aside, there are other reasons people don't buckle up. Myths have prevailed about seat belts ever since their first appearance in automobiles some 20 years ago. And the sooner those myths are set straight, the better. In talking with the experts, we've learned the following are most common.

MYTH 1: It's best to be "thrown clear" of a serious accident ● Sorry, but any accident serious enough to "throw you clear" is also going to be serious enough to give you a very bad landing. And chances are you'll have traveled through a windshield or door to do it. Studies show that chances of dying after an automobile accident are 25 times greater in cases where people are "thrown clear."

MYTH 2: Seat belts "trap" people in cars that are burning or sinking in water ● Sorry again, but studies show that people knocked unconscious due to *not* wearing seat belts have a greater chance of dying in accidents involving submersion or fire. People wearing belts usually are protected to the point of having sufficient wherewithal to free themselves from such emergencies, not be entrapped by them.

MYTH 3: Seat belts aren't needed at speeds of less than 30 mph ● In a head-on collision between two cars traveling at 30 mph, an unbelted driver would meet the windshield and dashboard with a force equal to diving headfirst into a sidewalk from three stories up. The body is given exactly a hundredth of a second to stop.

MYTH 4: Seat belts are more of a nuisance than anything else on short trips around home ● Studies show that fully 75 percent of all accidents occur within 25 miles of home—and that they happen at speeds of less than 40 mph. Deaths have been recorded at speeds as slow as 12 mph, the approximate velocity at which you might find yourself cruising the parking lot of your local supermarket.

MYTH 5: Most seat belts fit too loosely to work properly ●
The "play" in a seat belt is a feature (designed for comfort and ease of motion) that is quickly erased as soon as the belt is tugged on abruptly, as would be the case in the event of an accident. Hit your brakes hard some time if you're skeptical.

MYTH 6: Wearing a seat belt seems fatalistic ● No more fatalistic than the grim statistic that the average driver in this country can expect to be involved in a traffic accident at least once every ten years.

How to Buckle Up the Kids

At greatest danger of all in an automobile are small children. They don't have the strength (or sense) to brace themselves in emergency situations, and their bone structures are lighter and more susceptible to injury. They need special protection. How do you give it to them?

That depends on the size of the child. Children under 40 pounds or younger than four years should not be buckled up with standard lap belts, because the bones of a young pelvis simply are not strong enough to withstand a lap-belt's impact.

The best place for a car-bound little one is in his own specially designed car seat. There are many styles and brands available.

And don't think that just because a small child is being held in adult arms that he or she is safe. Even if the adult is buckled in, chances are slim that he'd be able to hold on to a child in the event of a serious mishap. And if the adult is not buckled in, he only becomes a potential squashing device.

In a word, *never* allow a small child to travel unrestrained in an automobile. Little ones might seem safe curled up asleep in a back seat or rear cargo area, but an unbuckled child is a potential missile in the event of even some fairly minor traffic mishaps. Be a good parent and always keep your kids well anchored.

So seat belts make sense. Immense sense. Studies leave no doubt that motor-vehicle fatalities could be reduced by 50 percent—and serious injuries by 65 percent—if we'd all simply buckle up.

But something else could be saved if we'd all buckle up: money. The National Highway Traffic Safety Administration estimates that society pays a whopping $40 billion a year in motor-vehicle crash costs. This amount could be significantly reduced if we'd all wear our seat belts.

So you're convinced seat belts make sense. And you're finally going to start wearing one. But are you going to let the buckle stop there?

Not if there are people in your life you care about. You might consider it your responsibility, in fact, to make the wisdom of seat belts known to people close to you, much the same as Elizabeth did with her dad. People are much more likely to listen to you because you *are* close to them, in fact.

The key to becoming a regular seat-belt user is to make it a habit, so take heart that you improve a person's chances of getting hooked on wearing a seat belt each and every time you get him to do it. With proper persuasion, those non-seat-belt-wearers in your life could soon feel downright naked without one.

How to Arrive Alive

Do you invest time and effort in maintaining a sound body? Good. What we want you to do is protect that investment when you slide behind the wheel of a car.

It's simply not enough that you obey the speed limit and wear your seat belt. Those are smart things to do. But safe driving demands something more.

Tuning Up the Driver

It doesn't matter that your car is in good shape if *you* aren't running on all eight cylinders.

Emotional stability is a crucial part of safe driving. What's more, people who aren't in control of their emotions are as much of a threat to themselves, other motorists and pedestrians as bad brakes or bald tires.

In one recent survey, one out of every five drivers killed in auto crashes had experienced some emotional upset within a six-hour period preceding the fatal accident.

There is such a thing as an accident-prone personality, according to Ming T. Tsuang, M.D., Ph.D., professor of psychiatry at the Harvard Medical School and chief of psychiatry at the Brockton-West Roxbury V.A. Medical Center.

It isn't difficult to spot this hot-tempered traffic hazard. Chances are, you know one. Among his chief defects, according to Dr. Tsuang: a hair-trigger temper, emotional immaturity and difficulty accepting authority.

Usually, such a person is unaware his personality puts himself or others at risk. Friends or spouse should point it out, says Dr. Tsuang. Once the accident-prone person is aware of his problem, adds Dr. Tsuang, "It is very important for him to learn not to get into the driver's seat when he is in a state of emotional turmoil, such as after an argument or when he is under some sort of stress."

There are other, far more obvious threats to your driving competence. Drinking, for one. Drugs, for another.

Either drugs or alcohol can interfere with your driving ability. What's new is that researchers have noticed a higher incidence of fatal accidents in which both alcohol and drugs were involved.

In California, researchers found that 10 percent of all fatally injured drivers showed evidence of diazepam, a tranquilizer, in their bloodstream. Of these, 70 percent also had been drinking.

Aside from mental or emotional limitations, there are physical driving limits, too. Vision problems are among the most serious, particularly for elderly motorists.

Many older people have trouble driving at night, for example. That's because the retina—the "film" in the back of the eye that receives outside images—doesn't respond as quickly to changes in light and dark. "Older drivers have difficulty dealing with headlight glare and they have trouble afterward readjusting to darkness," says Burt Skuza, O.D., executive director of the Minnesota Board of Optometry and chairman of the American Optometric Association's task force on older Americans.

If driving is a problem for you, Dr. Skuza offers a few words of advice. "I would try to stay off the road at rush hour," he recommends. "I would curtail or limit driving at night and try to do most of my driving during the daytime. Also, try to stay off the freeways, if at all possible."

Vision problems do make driving more risky. But problems also crop up in those of us who see just fine. That's because we don't always see what we think we see.

We reckon distances by visual angle—that is, we perceive large objects as close and small objects as far away. That was no problem when all cars were basically the same size—big. Not so any more. Cars may vary in width by as much as two feet.

So what does this mean to you? It means that you might be a lot closer to that small car than you think because you've misjudged its size. "People are so used to seeing larger cars that now that we have smaller cars, they think the small car is a larger car," according to Ray Eberts, Ph.D., assistant professor of industrial engineering at Purdue University.

What you need to do is become accustomed to looking for other visual cues. Obviously, if you're close enough to make out tiny details on the back of a car—like the name of the company that made the vehicle—you're too close. Also look for features like hatchbacks or yellow turn signals, both clues that the car you're following is a small car.

Driving after Dark

Overconfidence is your worst enemy after the sun goes down. "Fifty-seven percent of all collisions happen at night," says James Solomon, administrator of training for driver-improvement programs of the National Safety Council. "At night, you should slow down because not as much is visible to you as during the day. If you're on a dark country road, that's particularly true."

And don't be lulled into a false sense of security by those bright new quartz halogen headlights, either. "Most people have a tendency to overdrive their headlights," says Solomon. That is, even with the new headlights, driving at 35 mph, you still can see only about five seconds ahead of you. With standard headlights on low beam, your margin of safety is even lower.

One other hazard of nighttime driving is the seemingly oblivious "other guy" who drives with his high beams shining in your face. Most of us respond in kind, flicking our high beams on and off until he gets the message. But that's ineffective and potentially dangerous.

"The driver with the bright lights coming at you can be warning you of several things," advises Solomon. "He could be intoxicated. He could be driving a strange car and can't find the low beam switch. He could be elderly. His low beams could be out and he's trying to avoid the cops. Whatever you do, don't blink your high beams at him. All that's going to do is blind the person who is already having trouble operating his vehicle."

Here's what you should do instead:

● Move a little farther to the right.
● Look as far down the road in your lane as you can. The other guy's lights are probably illuminating that area for you.
● Concentrate the center of your vision toward the right side of the road.

Finally, before you drive at night, don't forget to clean the soot, salt and bugs off your headlights and turn-signal lights. Remember, headlights not only help you see better. They help the other guy see you, too.

Most of us worry about the road in bad weather. We're on the lookout for potholes and ice and such. Truth is, icy roads are dangerous, but most of us tend to compensate by driving more cautiously.

Contrary to what you might think, fair-weather driving can make for dangerous road conditions, too.

Remember that in warm weather, you're likely to encounter more traffic in unexpected places. There are garage sales, county fairs, tractors pulling farm equipment and volunteer firemen with their hats held out for donations.

Another hazard of summer, on asphalt roads, is oil. In intense summer heat, the oil in asphalt separates from the rest of the road material and rises to the surface, where it waits as a slippery surprise for the unwary driver, especially when it rains.

Get to Know Your Car

It makes sense to prepare your car for the coming season, to make certain it's in good running order and to be ready to handle a breakdown far from home or under hazardous weather conditions. But it's often the little things we overlook. For instance, do you really know the right way to use your sun visor?

Here's how. If you're driving into bright sunlight, pull the visor down and forward until it touches the windshield. Then pull it back toward you until it blocks the glare.

In other words, make certain the sharp edge of the visor is pointed *away* from your face. In an accident, your head could snap forward and the visor could cause a lot of damage to your forehead, your eyes or the bridge of your nose.

Another sun blocker is the tinted windshield. But for many of us, particularly older drivers, tinted glass also diminishes what little light is available at night. And that's a hazard.

If you have trouble seeing at night consider clear glass when you buy your next car, the American Optometric Association recommends.

How Not to Catch a Wave

When you drive in the rain, your tires push a wave of water ahead of them. At low speeds, this isn't much of a problem. But as you increase your speed— to 30 or 35 mph and higher—that wave can become a wedge between your tires and the road surface. This phenomenon is called hydroplaning.

Here are the telltale signs of hydroplaning:

● You try to turn the wheels, but the car keeps going forward.
● You hit the brakes, but get no response.
● In a front-wheel-drive car, you try to speed up, but you can't. Even though the wheels are turning faster, they aren't touching anything but water.

So what do you do?

First, *DO NOT* slam on the brakes. Second, "Ease off the gas," says James Solomon. "As the car slows, that wave starts to dissipate and the wheels start to touch the road again."

Heavy traffic almost demands that you be able to predict the future. You have to analyze what's happening up ahead and make an inspired guess as to what the other guy plans to do.

Police officers, who drive more than most of us do, have developed a few techniques of their own:

● *Scan 10 to 15 seconds ahead of you.* "Look beyond the car in front of you," advises Lt. Herbert Grofcsik, commanding officer of the driver-training unit at the Philadelphia Police Academy. "Two or three blocks is the minimum. If you're stuck behind a truck, stagger to the left a little bit and back again. As you go over a hill, expect something on the other side. Slow down."

● *Plan an escape route.* When you drive down the expressway, consider what you might do or where you would go if that propane truck coming up the ramp suddenly darted in front of you. Is there room on the shoulder? Is there oncoming traffic in the opposite lane? Is there a turning lane?

It's equally important to leave the other guy an escape route. So try not to drive for long periods alongside other cars, adds Lt. Grofcsik.

● *Wait three seconds after the light turns green.* Don't assume that all the traffic has cleared, says Lt. Grofcsik. The guy across from you might dart out to make a left turn in front of you. Drivers going in the other direction might try to beat the yellow light.

● *Try 3-9 steering.* Put your left hand at 9:00 your right hand at 3:00 on the steering wheel. This technique puts you in a better position to steer out of harm's way quickly, says Lt. Grofcsik.

If you're just making a normal turn, you can use the traditional hand-over-hand method. But if you have to turn quickly to evade something or someone that has stopped or run out in front of your car, keep your hands in the 3-9 position and turn the wheel sharply to the left. Your right arm will cross over your left arm. To get back, do the same thing in reverse until your hands are in the original position. And don't slam on the brakes. You'll probably skid into whatever it is you were trying to avoid.

Hints to Make a Long Drive Safer

There are other rules of the road that apply more to long drives:

● *Take the load off.* "On long trips, you should take a break from driving a minimum of once every two hours. Pull off the road at a rest stop, get out of the car and walk around," says the National Safety Council's James Solomon. "And if it's possible, switch driving with someone else."

● *Throw in the towel.* Solomon says over-the-road truckers commonly carry an insulated plastic bag filled with ice and a damp cloth. They use the cloth to wipe their faces every once in a while. It helps them stay alert.

● *Don't get too comfy.* Roll down the window and let in some air. "People tend to make their cars too comfortable," says Solomon. "On a long haul, you need a little bit of noise or a little bit of cool. Talking helps, too."

● *Listen to music you don't like . . .* If Frank Sinatra or Lionel Richie makes you swoon, find something more distracting. Or, Solomon suggests, try talk radio. Easy listening will rock you to sleep.

● *. . . but not too loud.* If you turn up the radio, it may effect your vision. Psychologists at Clarkson University in Potsdam, New York, found that when car stereos were cranked up high, drivers—college student volunteers, in this case—couldn't see as far or as well.

Learn how to be a better driver at night. For a free single brochure, "How to Drive after Dark," send a stamped, self-addressed long envelope with 37 cents postage, to: National Safety Council, Dept. PR-P, 444 N. Michigan Ave., Chicago, IL 60611. Be sure to request the brochure by name.

For older drivers, the American Optometric Association has prepared a special brochure, "Driving Tips for Older Adults." To get one free, send a stamped, self-addressed long envelope to: American Optometric Association, Communications Center-P, 243 N. Lindbergh Blvd., St. Louis, MO 63141.

You might also consider taking a defensive-driving course at your local chapter of the National Safety Council. In some states, taking a course may result in lower insurance rates or points off on your driving record.

Consult your telephone directory for the National Safety Council branch near you.

Index

Rodale Press, Inc., publishes PREVENTION®, the better health magazine.
For information on how to order your subscription,
write to PREVENTION®, Emmaus, PA 18049.